The Changing Federal Role in U.S. Health Care Policy

THE CHANGING FEDERAL ROLE IN U.S. HEALTH CARE POLICY

JENNIE JACOBS
KRONENFELD

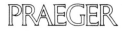

Westport, Connecticut
London

Library of Congress Cataloging-in-Publication Data

Kronenfeld, Jennie J.
    The changing federal role in U.S. health care policy / Jennie
Jacobs Kronenfeld.
        p. cm.
    Includes bibliographical references and index.
    ISBN 0-275-95023-9 (alk. paper). — ISBN 0-275-95024-7 (pbk. :
alk. paper)
    1. Medical policy—United States. 2. Medical care—United States.
3. Medical care—Law and legislation—United States. I. Title.
RA395.A3K757 1997
362.1'0973—dc21   97-19036

British Library Cataloguing in Publication Data is available.

Library of Congress Catalog Card Number: 97-19036
ISBN: 0-275-95023-9
        0-275-95024-7 (pbk.)

First published in 1997

Praeger Publishers, 88 Post Road West, Westport, CT 06881
An imprint of Greenwood Publishing Group, Inc.

Printed in the United States of America

∞™

The paper used in this book complies with the
Permanent Paper Standard issued by the National
Information Standards Organization (Z39.48-1984).

10 9 8 7 6 5 4 3 2 1

CONTENTS

Part II : The Federal Legislative
Process and Its Outcome

Part III: The Future of Health Care
and the Role of Government

Part I
The Evolving Federal Role in the U.S. Health Care System

1 GENERAL COMMENTS ON THE U.S. HEALTH CARE INFRASTRUCTURE AND DELIVERY SYSTEM

Health care in the United States at the end of the twentieth century occupies a completely different place in the economy, in the mind of the public, and in its impact on the government at all levels than it did either 100 years ago, at the beginning of the twentieth century, or at the beginning of the country in the late 1700s, when the U.S. Constitution was adopted. Health care in the United States is now a multibillion dollar industry, one that consumes 15 percent of the GDP (gross domestic product) of the country each year.

Moreover, that figure has been rising steadily over the past 30 years. The number of physicians, nurses, and other health care providers has increased to the point that some experts question whether the country has an oversupply. Modern hospitals have increased in size and complexity and have been described as modern temples of healing, although their role as the center of health care delivery is changing as the health care system itself changes. In fact, there are now questions whether the central role of the hospital as the linchpin and citadel of delivery of health care in the United States will hold as the new century begins (Stoeckle, 1995).

Citizens view health care as essential to their lives, and it is an unusual day when there are no articles in major national newspapers that relate to some aspect of health. Local television news shows run separate features on health care, because these are popular topics of discussion among their viewers. Most Americans today have grown accustomed to the medical miracles of penicillin and polio vaccines, as well as the rapid advances in the treatment of heart problems.

Many experts now agree that the U.S. health care system has had great successes, especially in the area of technology (Botelho, 1991; Todd, Seekins, Kirchbaum, and Harvey, 1991). The United States has achieved one of the most technologically advanced medical care systems in the world, and much of this technology is generally available to affluent and middle-class consumers of health care services. These achievements in technology are one of the reasons why the United States is now also an international leader in medical education, with physicians coming from all over the world both to receive the most advanced and sophisticated training, and to learn how to incorporate the newest equipment and technology into the practice of medicine (Todd et al., 1991).

This book focuses on the changing federal role in health care policy in the United States, and pays special attention to the changes in the Reagan-Bush years and the failed attempt at major health care reform during the first term of the Clinton presidency. Prior to a discussion of specific aspects of federal legislation and the role of the federal government in the delivery of health care, Part One of the book presents salient features of the U.S. health care system and its infrastructure. The first chapter focuses on more general comments about the system and perceptions of past and current problems, as well as the role of technology. Chapter 2 continues describing salient features of the U.S. health care system by exploring issues of costs of care, providers of care, and the increasing attention being paid to the development of a continuum of care. Part Two focuses on the federal legislative process and its outcomes, looking at the past as well as at the situation immediately prior to the election of President Clinton. One chapter focuses on the health policy process; another focuses on the history of federal involvement in health care and health policy, and upon basic federal health-related legislation through the Carter administration. The third chapter in this section focuses upon the Reagan and Bush years and the limited and reactive types of changes in health care policy at the national level that were enacted in that 12-year period, with greater focus on those more recent reforms. Part Three examines the current situation in health care policy, with a more detailed examination of the attempt at major health care reform in the first term of Clinton's presidency and various explanations for why that attempt failed. In the last chapter, the more modest changes in the health policy arena that were successfully passed during the initial term of the Clinton presidency are discussed, as is the issue of the future of health care in the United States and the role of government. This chapter also discusses how current health care issues and concerns may or may not set the stage for a changed federal role in funding and delivery of health care services in the next century.

THE CHANGING IMAGE OF A "CRISIS" IN HEALTH CARE

Despite the recognition of the advances in modern medicine and the important advances in medical technology and training for health care providers within the United States, most of the public does not necessarily view the U.S. health care system as perfect or as nonproblematic. In fact, public perceptions of health care overall and of the role of government in health care are fraught with recognition of diverse problems such as barriers to care, lack of health insurance for many people, and discussions of a "crisis" in health care delivery. The first two years of the Clinton presidency, and part of the political campaign leading up to that election in 1992, included wide public debate over health care and the proper role for the federal government in the provision and funding of health care services. Much of this debate was predicated on the question of whether there was a crisis in health care that necessitated comprehensive reform of our financing and delivery system. The failure of this campaign will be discussed in more detail in Chapter 6 of this book.

But the notion of a crisis—very important in the 1992 presidential election—partially arose from the results of the special senatorial election held in November 1991 to fill the Senate seat of Pennsylvania Senator John Heinz, who died in a plane crash in April 1991. In that campaign, Harris Wofford was the Democratic candidate for the Senate against the popular former governor of the state, Dick Thornburgh, the Republican candidate. Wofford made the issue of health care reform and improved access to health care a keystone of his campaign, and used many television spots stating, "If criminals have a right to a lawyer, I think working Americans should have the right to a doctor" (Johnson and Broder, 1996). In what was described by many political observers as a stunning upset, Wofford defeated Thornburgh by a 55 to 45 percent margin, setting the stage for a renewed focus on health care in the presidential campaign of 1992—first among the Democratic primary challengers, and then in the race of Clinton versus Bush in November 1992.

The Wofford-Thornburgh senatorial race was one example of recent open public discussion about a "crisis" in health care. These concerns about a crisis in U.S. health care are not new, however. Each decade for the past thirty years has been characterized by at least some discussion of a "health care crisis," making this a most overused phrase. The exact explanation for the health care crisis has varied over time, from a crisis of access and affordable care for the elderly in the 1960s (which was partially resolved by the creation of the Medicare program), to a crisis of rapidly rising costs in the 1970s and 1980s, to crises about lack of enough generalist physicians and lack of health care in rural areas, among many other possible sources of problems.

Certainly a major crisis that has been discussed for decades is the issue of access to health care services, and suggestions for the resolution to this crisis have often involved government, at the same time, and have frequently included the opposition of some health and medical groups. The Committee on the Costs of Medical Care was created in the late 1920s, on the eve of the Depression. Its report called for a massive reorganization of the fee-for-service medical care system, and urged some version of national health insurance. When the committee report was issued in the fall of 1932, the American Medical Association (AMA, the largest association of physicians of various specialties across the United States) condemned the report and raised such fierce opposition that Franklin Roosevelt was forced to remove medical benefits from his first Social Security bill (Johnson and Broder, 1996; Starr, 1982). By 1943, during World War II, liberal Democrats with the backing of organized labor introduced the first compulsory national health insurance bill. Both the preoccupation of President Roosevelt and the continued opposition of the AMA, joined this time by the nation's pharmaceutical and insurance industries, led to the defeat of this legislation (Johnson and Broder, 1996).

A few years later, President Truman introduced health insurance legislation and made its lack of enactment a major issue in the 1948 presidential campaign. After Truman's upset victory, the AMA launched a major campaign against a national health insurance bill, warning that such legislation would lead to federal control of health care. The AMA again lined up powerful allies, including groups outside the health care industry such as the U.S. Chamber of Commerce and the American Farm Bureau.

One effort that actually led to major federal legislation was the passage of Medicare and Medicaid in 1965. Although the AMA continued its tradition of opposition to any major government role in paying for or providing health care services, the landslide victory of Lyndon Johnson over Barry Goldwater, creating large Democratic majorities in both the House and the Senate, was responsible for the passage of this major legislation that dramatically increased access to health care for the elderly and the poor in the United States.

Although various more modest pieces of legislation were passed in the United States in the decades following 1965, most did not focus on access to care. By May 1991, the AMA and many other health groups had become convinced about the growing importance of the problem of access. In that year, the Journal of the American Medical Association (JAMA), as well as the specialty publications of the AMA, published special issues focused on caring for the uninsured and underinsured. One of the articles pointed out that a national commission on medical and ethical problems in 1983 had concluded that society has a moral obligation to ensure that everyone in the United States has access to adequate medical care (Menken, 1991; President's Commission, 1983). By this standard, the author concluded that the health system of the United States is failing. One major policy question is whether there is a public consensus that the conclusions of the commission (that everyone should have access to adequate health care) are correct. Even if there is a public consensus that everyone should have access to adequate health care, a further issue is the definition of "adequate."

While such definitions differ, most agree that having no health care insurance makes a person much less likely to be able to afford needed health care services. Although estimates of the number of those uninsured in the United States vary slightly from one expert to another, and change somewhat from year to year, many experts agree that from 33 to 40 million Americans are uninsured and are thus, at times, unable to receive needed health care services. Many of these people without health insurance are currently working—but in jobs that do not provide health care insurance coverage. Some of the others are family members of working people, whose employers provide insurance coverage only for the employee, with no option for family members.

Another way to think about definitions of adequate care is to compare what people in America spend versus those in other countries. In this area, as a nation, the United States is a large spender for health care services. The United States spent more per capita on health care in 1994 than did any of the other 26 richest nations in the world. In that year, U.S. spending on health care was $3,516 per capita, or 14.3 percent of the gross domestic product (GDP). The next closest nation to the spending patterns in the United States was Switzerland, which spent 9.6 percent of GDP, or $2,294 per person (Montague, 1996).

Public opinion polling data, as well as general discussion of social and health care issues in the society, both provide evidence that the public consensus on this problem has changed just over the decade of the 1990s. Before discussing the changing views of the role of government in health care that the public has held, as well as specific issues such as technology, costs of care, and the growth of different methods and approaches for the delivery and receipt of health care services, it is helpful to cover some major aspects of the current system of health care in the United States. Included in this discussion is a brief contrast between the system in the United States and the systems in selected other countries.

PRIMARY, SECONDARY, AND TERTIARY CARE AND LINKAGES TO REGIONALIZED VERSUS DISPERSED MODELS

One classic description of systems of health care involves the distinction among primary, secondary, and tertiary levels of care (Dawson, 1975; Grumbach and Bodenheimer, 1995). Primary care involves treatment for most common health problems, as well as preventive care. Examples of common ailments would include sore throats, sprained wrists, and infected ears. Screening for hypertension, and vaccinating babies and children are examples of preventive care. Secondary care is that provided for more specialized problems and would include surgery to set a broken leg, or care for an older patient who develops acute renal failure. Tertiary care is reserved for the most specialized and unusual health care problems; it is not the type of care that can be provided by most full-service hospitals, but rather it is care that different specialty facilities may provide. Thus, in one city, there may be a hospital that provides open-heart surgery as the most advanced, newest treatment, while a different facility may provide the setting and most accessible equipment for neurosurgery. In a different city, a university hospital may well provide a complete range of tertiary care.

An understanding of these three different levels of care helps in describing contrasting models for the delivery of health care, both at a national and at a local level. One often-discussed distinction is that between a regionalized model of care versus a dispersed model of care (Grumbach and Bodenheimer, 1995). One model that can be used is based at a national level on regionalization and at a community-wide level on a distinction between a person's usual, more typical care versus the need for more specialized services. In this regionalized system, personnel and facilities will be differentially assigned to tiers of care that correspond to the primary-secondary-tertiary care structure (Grumbach and Bodenheimer, 1995). Patients will flow across the levels of care as needs dictate.

While the health care systems in most countries often embody elements of both models, some countries' systems more closely resemble one or the other. The model of regionalization closely resembles the organization used by the British National Health Service (and does not resemble the model for health care overall in the United States at present). Many other countries, such as those in Scandinavia and some of the developing nations in Latin America, have adopted this type of approach to the delivery of health care services.

At a more community-based level, the model is applied by some health maintenance organizations (HMOs) within the United States, especially those that operate with a closed panel of physicians who work full-time for the plan in a group practice approach. In those types of HMOs, patients must obtain all of their care from within the closed panel of physicians, and they generally begin with a generalist physician who provides the primary level of care and some limited secondary care. Within the same building, there may be some specialists with the plan who provide some types of secondary care. More complicated secondary and tertiary care will be referred to other physicians within the plan, or, in some cases, to outside physicians who contract with the group for the most advanced tertiary care.

The alternative model of care is often described as a dispersed model (Grumbach and Bodenheimer, 1995), which gives greater choice to patients and caregivers, whether it is applied at a national or local level. Within a national level of care, this model describes a system without explicit regionalization, so that one community may have five different facilities providing highly technical specialized care (such as the newest procedures to treat heart disease, for example) in contrast to a community probably having only one or two such centers in a regionalized model. In fact, in the regionalized model, many smaller towns and rural areas would not have any tertiary care available within the community, with probably only the more general secondary care. In the dispersed model, if a community could generate enough funds and attract the appropriate physician, a small town might still have available more advanced cardiac services, for example. At the community-wide level, the dispersed model allows patients to pick for themselves among various providers of care. It also allows providers greater freedom, in that they are generally able to refer to other specialists as they see the need develop, and to use for referrals a physician or group of physicians with whom they have developed a professional relationship, whether or not any special payment and fee arrangements have been worked out.

This alternative or dispersed model is a better description of the current operation of the U.S. health care system overall. It also describes best how patients who are not part of managed care or HMO models in the United States obtain their health care services within the community in which they live. The dispersed model thus represents the way most people in the United States have obtained their health care in the past, although, given the growth of managed care, more people are beginning to experience a model of care that incorporates some elements of the regionalization model. In the dispersed model, patients are not required to have a primary care physician who must make decisions about seeking care at higher levels, which is the way the regionalized model operates in Great Britain and the way some HMOs operate within the United States.

Is one of these models a better or more appropriate way to deliver health care services? Critiques of both approaches exist. Critics of the dispersed model, which has formed the basis for the traditional delivery of health care in the United States, argue that the system is top-heavy, with too many specialists and too few generalists. Related to this is the criticism that the U.S. system provides a focus on more advanced levels of care and tertiary facilities, rather than a focus on primary care. However, most people need primary and simpler levels of services most of the time, and these can be provided by generalists. Another criticism of the U.S. system is the lack of a clear organizational structure. How patients are supposed to figure out what type of physician to go to first, and where to find this physician, is often unclear in the dispersed model. Moreover, a patient may consult several physicians about different problems at the same time, and if the patient does not think or remember to discuss this with the second or third physician, each may be unaware that the patient is currently undergoing treatment by a colleague. A physician could even prescribe a drug for one problem that could interfere with, or be dangerous when taken with, a drug prescribed by a different physician for a separate problem. This issue has often been described as a lack of continuity and coordination in care (Kronenfeld, 1980). Torrens (1993) describes this aspect of the private-practice, fee-for-service system of health care in the United States as an informal system, in which there is an absence of any defined structure or organization to create continuity of care across time and across provider.

Advocates of the dispersed model that has been an important traditional approach to the delivery of health care in the United States argue that pluralism is a virtue, because it promotes flexibility and convenience in the availability of personnel and facilities (Grumback and Bodenheimer, 1995). The emphasis on specialization and technology is viewed as particularly congruent with American values and expectations, since Americans prefer choice in many areas and value technology greatly. In many areas of American life, people prefer the best, the most advanced, and the newest. One way Americans have been able to actualize these preferences in the health care system has been through a dispersed model of care, even if it has led to higher costs and a less easily understood system for obtaining health care.

Critics of the regionalized model of care are fearful that such a model removes too many choices from patients and places too much power in the hands of those who determine how to regionalize the system—whether these are executives of managed care programs in HMOs within the United States or bureaucrats in a government agency. With the growth of HMOs and managed care organizations in the United States in the last five years, there has been a growth of consumer complaints about denials of care. These include denials of newer medications, denials of certain newer treatments, and denied permission to see specialists. If this model becomes more common, these complaints may proliferate and some remedies may have to be found, perhaps in greater government regulation of the managed care companies.

A more important fear about a regionalized model in the United States, which became one factor in concerns about the Clinton reform plan that was not passed in 1993–94, is that government will hold too much power over the fates of individuals. Within the United States, this concern fits neatly into one cultural paradigm of concern about "big" government and a feeling that the best government is small and at a level close to the individual. The specter of a large national health insurance agency making decisions about which doctor a patient can go to and what treatment he or she can receive touches upon pivotal American concerns about autonomy, self-control, and freedom of choice of provider and treatment. It also raises American fears about "Big Brother," who will know too much about intimate details of the life of an individual if health care information is centralized in a large, federal bureaucracy. Moreover, the last several decades—and especially the Reagan years—have heightened the traditional American dislike of bureaucracy and created a public image of inefficient government agencies that cannot be trusted with major control over the most important aspects of a person's life. Because at times of the most serious illnesses, access to the best health care often becomes a "life or death" issue, emotions about such access being controlled by government touch many of the deepest fears of some Americans.

Advocates of a regionalized model argue that it would better help to define practitioner roles, which might lead to a more appropriate split between specialization and primary care among American physicians, a problem of long standing in the American health care system. Proponents of this model also argue that it would increase the accountability of care for the whole patient, and thus ultimately have the potential to improve the total quality of care that patients receive, since there would be a generalist physician overseeing the total provision of care.

TECHNOLOGY AND CARE

The preeminence of the dispersed model of care in the United States during the twentieth century is linked with 1) the preeminence of the biomedical model among physicians and others within the health care system, 2) the preeminence of medicine in the United States compared to many other countries in the post-World War II years, and 3) the importance placed upon technology and the development of new technology. To understand the problems of the U.S. health care system today, as well as issues that will have to be addressed in the future either by the federal government or by market-driven reorganization of care, a better appreciation of the role of technology within health care in the United States is important.

In the early twentieth century, the biomedical model became the dominant approach for the education of physicians in the United States (Starr, 1982; Grumback and Bodenheimer, 1995). Part of the push toward the adoption of a biomedical model was a result of the impact of the Flexner Report in 1910, which pointed out great deficiencies in medical education in the United States at that time. These deficiencies included a lack of science background for entering students and the absence of both laboratory science and direct clinical education for medical students. Many existing medical schools subsequently closed, and most of those remaining in operation, as well as new ones begun after the Flexner Report, became affiliated with universities and began to hire faculty that were scientific investigators as well as clinicians (Starr, 1982; Stevens, 1971). Academic medical centers thus embraced the biomedical paradigm that was the outgrowth of the success of such European micro-biologists as Pasteur and Koch—with their famous discoveries leading to pasteurization of milk, treatment for rabies, and identification of the bacillus that causes tuberculosis. Related to this approach is the concept that every illness has a discrete and knowable cause, with the resultant concept of "magic bullets" that can cure an illness, as the knowledge of sources of disease increases. From this biomedical model came the emphasis on specialization, with physicians learning to understand the pathophysiology of particular organ systems. Part of this biomedical approach and focus on medicine as more of a science and less of the art of an earlier period led away from a recognition of patients as people, embedded within a family, community, and broader social system, and away from seeing the patient as a whole human being, rather than as a collection of organ systems.

Several different factors have contributed to the preeminence of U.S. medicine in the last forty years. One of these is the advantage of a sup-portive medical infrastructure. Not all of this is linked to the federal gov-ernment, although it has played a very important role in the funding of research. Some research is conducted with nonfederal funds: pharmaceu-tical and medical equipment companies have helped to conduct medical research. High private funding levels for medical research and technology development have contributed to the stature of U.S. medicine. And before this decade, medical research received wide public support and funding levels from the federal government that matched that wide support.

Support for the development of new technology has a long tradition in American society, not only in medicine. The United States was settled by individuals who were pragmatic and often antiintellectual, placing a value on tools and equipment over abstract knowledge. While the inventiveness of which Americans were proud was generally self-funded or part of indus-try prior to the twentieth century, inventors such as Thomas Edison, Henry Ford, and Samuel Morse became folk heroes within American culture. Technological innovation became revered as a worthy goal in its own right. The field of medicine in the United States has not been immune to this American love affair with technology; rather, medicine has adopted tech-nology as part of its essential character. Many new inventions in medical technology and new treatments have been developed and adopted first in the United States. American medicine adopts new technology and approaches to treatment more rapidly than the medical establishment in other countries—both as a result of the cultural acceptability and because the presence of a dispersed model of care and many specialists has facili-tated the rapid spread of technology compared to a controlled pattern of introduction of innovation in more regionalized systems of care. Thus the decentralization of U.S. research and development has facilitated innovation and technological advances in medicine.

PUBLIC OPINION AND HEALTH CARE ACCESS

What does the public believe about health care? What does the public believe about government and how well it works? And what if one combines these issues? Much of this book deals with the interaction between the public (as the ultimate decision makers in a democratic form of government) and the health care system. Over the years, there have been many debates about what basic rights a society owes to any citizen. While different people often arrive at different answers to this question, one factor that distinguishes the United States from other industrialized countries is the lack of clarity as to whether the United States regards health care access as a basic human right (Davis, Gold, and Maleac, 1981; Friedman, 1991; Mullan, 1987). In almost all other countries, a citizen who becomes ill does have a right to receive some health care services, and often the services to which a person is entitled are quite comprehensive. Not all countries achieve this with the same type of health care system. While some countries have a true national health care service, such as the system in Great Britain mentioned in an earlier section of this chapter, others have a much more complex system that often is composed of different health insurance mechanisms. While these may appear to have some similarity to the system in the United States, the difference is that in these other countries people who are ill or worried about their health have a fairly clear mechanism by which to receive initial health care. While, depending upon the problem, a person might have to wait for treatment or even be told that the newest technology that might be available to wealthy, well-insured individuals in the United States is not currently available, most experts feel that coverage for basic care is more complete and simpler to obtain in most other countries than it is in the United States.

Does the United States view health care as a basic right? How does the concept of equity relate to any presumed right to health care? These are complex issues; moreover, the notion of equity is applicable to other areas of services in modern societies, such as education, as well as to health care (Kronenfeld, 1993). Is the goal of a just society the equal opportunity to achieve or is it to acquire equivalent results? One complexity in health care is the wide physiological and genetic variability in health. Two coexistent, but contradictory, traditions in the United States influence view on access to services, especially health care services. One tradition holds that individuals are responsible for their own welfare, including health care. The other tradition contends that communities have a responsibility to provide access to health care for all citizens, with a special concern about those unable to secure access on their own.

Who currently has access to health care in the United States? The employment–insurance link is the organizational backbone of our health insurance system, combined with Medicare for the elderly and Medicaid for the poor and for specialized types of services for some elderly (especially nursing home care). Most working-age Americans receive their health insurance coverage through their jobs or their spouse's jobs (Ruttenberg, 1994). The present system of employer-sponsored health insurance became common after the defeat of national health insurance proposals in the Truman administration in the late 1940s. These coverage plans were available in some industries sooner, because one of the reactions to wage controls in place during World War II was to provide new benefits to workers as a way to attract and retain employees. During that period, fringe benefits providing up to 5 percent of wages were not considered inflationary. Total enrollment in group hospital plans increased from less than 7 million at the beginning of World War II to 26 million people, covering a fifth of the population. By 1954, over 60 percent of the population had some form of hospital insurance, although coverage for medical services was much more limited (Anderson and Feldman, 1956).

Later, in 1961, changes in the federal tax code made health insurance packages to employees even more attractive by allowing employers' contributions to the plans to count as wages and be deducted as expenses (Jecker, 1994). Today, workplace health insurance is the dominant form of private health insurance. While coverage continued to increase in the 1960s and 1970s (and government programs to cover others also increased), the numbers of uninsured and underinsured have steadily increased since the late 1970s. At that time, the best estimates were that 25 to 26 million people in the United States were without health insurance. This amounted to 13 percent of the population under the age of 65 (the age at which most people become covered by the federal Medicare program). The numbers of uninsured grew in the 1980s, and by 1992, estimates ranged from a low of 22 million to a high of 37 million, with some more recent estimates closer to 40 million Americans that are not covered by private health insurance or government programs. Included in those with no coverage are people temporarily out of work, those who work for companies that do not provide coverage (most typically service industries and low-wage jobs) and those such as the homeless who are currently experiencing major social dislocations. Since about 85 percent of all private coverage is purchased through the workplace, one major factor in the increase in the number of uninsured in the 1980s was the growth in unemployment at that time and again in the early 1990s. The numbers of uninsured have not been returning to lower levels as unemployment rates have improved. One explanation for this may be the shift in types of employment, such as movement away from manufacturing jobs that typically provided comprehensive health insurance benefits to service jobs that often provide no health insurance or limited types of coverages.

The attitudes of the public toward health care, needed changes in health care, and how well providers and health care facilities are performing in American society change at various points. Later chapters of this book will focus in more detail on changes in public attitudes that occurred during the health care debate of 1993–94 and which contributed to the failure of the Clinton health care reform plan. The rest of this chapter focuses on more general public attitudes about health care, government, and the notion of "the health care crisis."

Support for health care reform of some type, as well as for expanding access to health care services for many Americans, is not new. Nor is general satisfaction with many aspects of health care. The Robert Wood Johnson Foundation conducted several special studies about access to health care and attitudes about health care in the United States in the late 1970s and 1980s (Access to Health Care in the United States, 1987; A New Survey on Access to Medical Care, 1978; Updated Report on Access to Health Care for the American People, 1983). In 1986, about three-quarters of those surveyed were satisfied with their most recent hospital visits, and even more (about 83 percent) were satisfied with their most recent ambulatory visits. These figures were very similar to those in the earlier survey completed in 1983 and similar to those from the earliest study by the RWJ Foundation.

Support for some type of national health insurance has been common in public opinion polls for the last twenty years. Figures do change some over time, however, and support for national health insurance reached a forty-year high of 66 percent in 1992 (Blendon, Brodie, and Benson, 1995a). In that same election year of 1992, voters ranked health care as the third most important factor in their presidential choice, behind only the economy and the federal budget deficit. The 1992 period also was a high point for Americans to feel there was a health care crisis, with 90 percent of those interviewed in May 1993 surveys stating there was a crisis (Blendon, Altman, Benson, Brodie, James, and Chervinsky, 1995b).

These attitudes were not simple, however, and were based on how people felt about their own health care situations and whether they thought the kind of health care reforms being suggested during the 1992 presidential election and during the early part of the Clinton administration push for health care reform would be good for them personally (Blendon et al., 1995a). The strong support for some type of reform in national health care declined if the questions implied that personal sacrifices would be required. Decline in support was particularly strong if people believed that health care reform would limit their own choice of doctors, require rationing, or reduce the current quality of care.

One explanation for these declines in support for health care reform if people thought their own care would be threatened was the generally cynical view that most Americans held toward government. Trust in government and the belief that the government would do the appropriate things at the times of policy decisions have changed over the last 40 years. In the mid 1960s, when Lyndon Johnson was president and Medicare and Medicaid were enacted as major health care reforms that expanded the role of the federal government as a direct payer for health care, 69 percent of Americans said they trusted the federal government to do what is right most of the time. By March 1993, when the Clinton administration was working on its health care reform plan, only 23 percent of the public expressed this level of trust. In contrast, attitudes of suspicion toward the government were fairly high. About 65 percent of the population reported that the federal government controlled too much of their daily lives; 69 percent reported that, when something is run by the government, it is usually inefficient and wasteful; and 80 percent said that the value they get from their taxes paid to the federal government was only fair or poor. Perhaps most negative in terms of the chances for enactment of a major expansion in the role of the federal government in health care, 60 percent favored a smaller government with fewer services (Blendon et al., 1995a).

At the time of the debate about health care reform in 1992 and the ensuing presidential election, this notion of a crisis in health care was supported by much of the public in systematic opinion polling. This was despite articles in the press arguing that uninsured citizens were not being denied health care, and that it was only a very small proportion of the population that was unable to obtain affordable health insurance (about 3 percent according to one article in the *Wall Street Journal*) (Stelzer, 1994). How have these opinions changed in the last few years? What do these changing opinions say to leadership in health care, whether governmental leaders or those involved in the direct delivery of health care services?

The Henry J. Kaiser Foundation has funded some new studies of public opinion about health insurance and access to health care. Almost 4000 telephone interviews were conducted from February through April of 1995 (Donelan, Blendon, Hill, Hoffmack, Rowland, Frankel, and Altman, 1996). About 18 percent of those surveyed reported there was a time in the past year when they did not get medical care that they thought they needed. A similar percentage (16 percent) reported that they had a problem in the last year in paying for their medical care bills. During the year of the survey, 19 percent of the people were without health care insurance either for the entire year (12 percent) or at some point in the year (7 percent). One's view of the health care system varies a great deal depending upon whether health care insurance is in force or not. The uninsured were four times more likely than the insured to report an episode of needing care and not getting it, and three times more likely to report a problem in paying for medical care bills.

Who in 1995 were the uninsured? Most (70 percent) were working at least part of the year, and 40 percent worked for employers who did provide health insurance coverage to some employees. The two main reasons the uninsured did not have health insurance were costs of the insurance and the lack of its availability through their employment (Donelan et al., 1996).

Do people receive care when they need it? Forty-five percent of the uninsured and 11 percent of the insured reported a time in the year prior to the survey when they were unable to obtain care. Almost a third of those who reported themselves in fair to poor health or as having a disability also reported a time of not receiving care. Cost and lack of insurance were the prime reasons people did not receive care. While many in this country think that the uninsured are able to receive charity or free care if they need it, the respondents to this survey did not find this to be the case most of the time. Only 37 percent of the uninsured who reported problems paying medical bills had received any free or reduced-charge care in the past year. Many were paying substantial amounts of money for health care. Among the uninsured, half had spent over $1000 in medical bills in the year prior to the survey and 8 percent had spent over $5000. Problems in paying medical bills occur even for those with health care insurance. Earlier studies have reported that, in 1992, 19 percent of Americans had problems in paying medical bills, and 75 percent of those were people with health care insurance (Blendon, Donelan, Hill, Carter, Beatrice, and Altman, 1994). In 1995, 58 percent of people with problems in paying medical bills were insured for the whole year and another 14 percent were insured for at least part of the year prior to the survey. The reasons that people had problems with costs despite having health insurance were linked with co-payments, deductibles, and coinsurance requirements, as well as with needing services not covered by the health insurance plan.

These survey results can be explained in several different ways, perhaps linked to the old adage of whether a person views a glass as half empty or half full. One interpretation is that most people have health insurance, receive care when they need it, and do not find the costs of either health insurance or health care to be burdensome. This is the good news, the half-full glass explanation. The other interpretation is that 50 million adults in this survey experienced difficulty receiving care in the past year, and that 34 million felt these problems were serious and could have an impact upon their future health.

How these different opinions are translated into either changes in or continuation of the health care system is a complex topic. How the problems that people experience link to both overall expenditures for health care and changes in the ways people receive care are also complex. The next chapter describes more about how the U.S. health care infrastructure works currently, with a focus upon costs of care, providers of care, and the changing structure of care. Part Two focuses more upon the federal role, looking at how political factors influence health policy, and the major federal roles in building the health care infrastructure and providing access to health care in the United States. Included in that section are chapters reviewing the major overall structure of federal health legislation and a chapter reviewing in more detail the changes during the Reagan and Bush years, 1980 through 1991. Part Three focuses upon the recent past, present, and speculations about the future. Chapter 6 focuses upon the failed attempts during the initial Clinton term to enact major health care reform at the federal government level. The last chapter reviews remaining problems and the potential for future health care reform, a potential linked to the attitudes and problems reported by the public in the recent Kaiser Foundation survey (Donelan et al., 1996).

2 SALIENT FEATURES OF THE U.S. HEALTH CARE INFRASTRUCTURE AND DELIVERY SYSTEM

This chapter will discuss three major issues in the U.S. health care delivery system and its infrastructure: costs of care, providers of care, and the continuum of care. The section on costs of care includes a consideration of how many dollars the country is spending for health care, how allocation of these costs has been changing over time, and major efforts to control costs of health care. Given the focus of the book on the federal role in the delivery of health care, another important issue is the extent to which government funds are being used for health care costs and how this has changed over time.

The second issue in this chapter involves review of some material about providers of care, who they are and the important issues. This information will provide background so that details of federal policy about providers—both individuals and institutions—that are discussed in the second part of this book can be understood within the broader context of relevant issues in the U.S. health care system today.

The concluding section presents the broadened perspectives of what care means and covers today. One term that is used (although often with a more narrow meaning than that proposed in this book) is the continuum of care. Some writers apply this term mostly to the elderly and links the stages of care as one develops serious illnesses and moves from hospital to home care to nursing home care. However, this book will use the term more broadly to cover a whole range of potential services from prevention to acute care. The range encompasses 1) primary care as described in Chapter 1, to 2) more advanced types of services such as are provided in a hospital, to 3) the types of services that may be required either as part of a rehabilitation process or as part of the end of life, such as home health care services, nursing home care, and hospice care.

COSTS OF CARE

One useful approach used by many analysts of our health care financing system is to talk about four categories of expenses: how much money is spent, where the money comes from (direct out-of-pocket, private insurance, government), what it is spent on (fees paid to individual providers, to hospitals, for drugs or medically-related supplies) and how it is paid out to the providers (per unit of service, per item of care, per hospital discharge, per day of long-term care services) (Jonas, 1992). Although the following discussion will not adhere strictly to these categorizations, they present a useful way to summarize one aspect of financing of health care services.

Trends in Health Care Expenditures

Rising health care costs have been an important factor in the health care system, from the 1940s up to the 1990s. During the 1990s, growth in health care costs has slowed considerably, although concern about costs continues (Cowan, Braden, McDonnell, and Sivarajan, 1996). National health care expenditures have grown at a rate substantially outpacing the gross national product (GNP) in most years since 1940. Prior to World War II, only 4 percent of the GNP was spent on health care. By 1960, this figure had increased only to 5.3 percent. Expressed in per capita terms, the growth in health expenditures appears much larger, partially because this was a period of rapid economic growth. Per capita expenses increased from $30 per capita in 1940 to $146 in 1960 (Waldo, Levit, and Lazerby, 1986).

These trends continued and accelerated in the next decades, as can be understood by comparing figures from 1960 to 1990 and beyond. The percent of GNP spent on health care increased to 7.4 percent in 1970 and 9.4 percent in 1980. Per capita expenses also continued to increase, going from $350 in 1970 to $1049 in 1980 in constant dollars (Waldo, et al., 1986). These trends are illustrated in Figure 2-1.

These decade-long figures actually mask important trends occurring within each decade. Health expenditures as a percentage of GNP were quite stable from 1950 to 1955, with more increase in the latter part of that decade (Kronenfeld and Whicker, 1984). Major impacts on expenditures were created by the passage of Medicare and Medicaid in 1965 and the beginning operation of those programs in 1966 (those figures will be examined in more detail shortly). A period of stabilization of prices occurred from 1971 to 1973 because the federal government had wage and price controls in place due to the Economic Stabilization Program (ESP) (Levit, Lazerby, Letsch, and Cowan, 1991a). After the lifting of all ESP controls and the expansion of the

Figure 2-1 *Percent Growth in National Health Expenditures and Gross Domestic Product, and National Health Expenditures as a Percentage of Gross Domestic Product: Calendar Years: 1960–94*

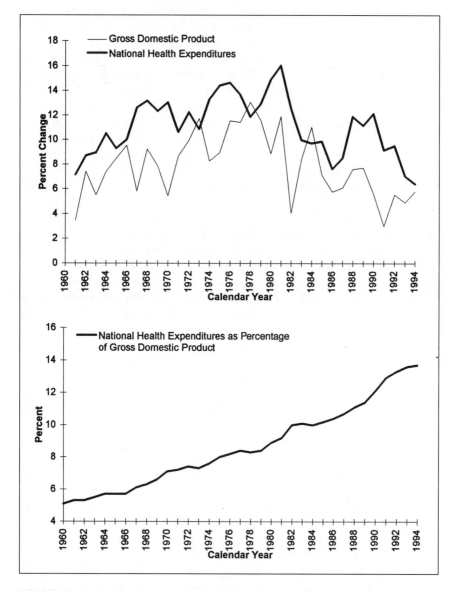

SOURCE: Health Care Financing Administration, Office of the Actuary: Data from the Office of National Health Statistics.

Medicare program to include the disabled more completely, costs rose to 8.5 percent of GNP by 1976. Then a voluntary effort to hold down health care costs ensued from 1976 through 1979 but gradually lost its effectiveness.

What has happened to health care expenditures during the decade of the 1980s and the first half of the 1990s? During the 1980s, pressures continued to build overall, despite various efforts to control spending and hold down costs in certain sectors—such as the passage of the DRG (diagnostic related groups) payment system for Medicare hospital expenses in the early 1980s. Spending for health care continued to grow by almost all measures, with particular acceleration from 1986 to the early 1990s (Lazerby and Letsch, 1990). By 1990, health care expenditures reached $666.2 billion, up to 12.2 percent of the gross national product and an increase of 10.5 percent from 1989 to 1990. This was an inflation rate substantially greater than the increase in overall GNP. In fact, the increase in the share of GNP spent for health care from 1989 to 1990 was the second largest such jump since 1960. The percentage of the GNP being expended on health care had increased to 10.7 percent in 1985, 11.6 percent in 1989, and 12.2 percent in 1990 (Levit, Lazerby, Cowan, and Letsch, 1991b). One explanation for the large jump was the slowdown in the general economy. Percentage of GNP spent on health is sensitive to overall economic growth because the denominator figure in percentage of GNP spent on health is a measure of overall output of the economy.

The trends in per capita expenditure are less dependent on overall economic trends. Per capita expenditures also continued to increase, up to $2,354 per capita in 1989 and $2,566 in 1990. This was an increase of 9.4 percent in one year. Of these per capita expenditures, public funds accounted for $1,089 per capita (42.4 percent of the total expenditures for health care) and private funds paid for the remaining $1,478 (57.6 percent) (Levit et al., 1991b).

After nearly five years of double-digit or near double-digit growth in aggregate health spending between 1988 and 1992, health care expenditure growth decelerated to 7 percent in 1993 and 6.4 percent in 1994 (Levit, Lazerby, Sivarajan, Stewart, Braden, Cowan, Donham, Long, McDonnell, Sensenig, Stiller, and Won, 1996b). The actual increase in health care dollars spent (now generally reported as a proportion of the GDP, gross domestic product) led to only a small increase in health care spending as a proportion of GDP from 13.6 percent in 1993 to 13.7 percent in 1994 (Levit et al., 1996b). One way to interpret this slower growth in health expenditures is to relate it to real or inflation-adjusted national health expenditures (NHE). When economy-wide inflation is removed from NHE, by using a chain-type annual weighted price index (Landerfeld and Parker, 1995), results measure the value of health care purchases in terms of the forgone opportunities to purchase other goods and services. In 1994, real NHE grew 4 percent, as additional purchases of health care were substituted for other goods and services. The runaway health care expenditures measured from 1988 to 1992 had subsided. A cautionary note is that two years does not make a true trend, and some experts believe that the current lowered costs are a reaction to threats of greater governmental involvement resulting from the failed health reform effort in 1993–94. Whether these trends of lowered increases in costs will continue throughout the 1990s and into the twenty-first century is not at all certain.

Trends in Types of Health Care Expenditures and Sources of Funds

Figure 2-2 shows both the sources of the nation's health dollars and where they went, in 1960 and in 1994, the most recent year for which data are available from the Health Care Financing Administration (HCFA), the federal agency that administers the Medicare and Medicaid programs and organizes much of the national data on health care spending. This provides a comparison of sources of revenue and expenditure over time, before beginning a more detailed examination first of types of health care expenditures and then of sources of revenue. A comparison of the sources of funds between 1960 and 1994 shows the greater influence of the role of government by 1994. Only 24 cents out of every health dollar in 1960 came from government programs. By 1994, government programs of all types provided 45 cents out of each health dollar—18 cents for Medicare, 14 for Medicaid (neither of which existed as a separate program in 1960), and the rest for other types of government programs both at the federal level and at state and local levels. The next largest source of the health care dollar in 1994 was private health insurance, which covered 33 cents. In 1960, private health insurance covered only 22 cents of each dollar. Far and away the largest source of the health care dollar in 1960 was out-of-pocket payments (that is, costs not reimbursed to the consumer). This category comprised 49 cents, or almost half of each health care dollar, in 1960 but comprised only 18 cents by 1994.

A comparison of where the health care dollar actually went in 1960 and 1994 reveals marked similarities over the 34 years. Hospital care was the largest single category of expense at both times, and took up 34 cents of the health care dollar in 1960 and 36 cents in 1994. The emphasis on hospital care has changed over the last five years: the amount of the health care dollar spent on hospital services was actually higher in 1990, 38 cents. This reflects a decline in the importance of hospital care within the overall continuum of care, a trend discussed more in the second and third portions of this chapter.

The catch-all category of other personal health care, which includes such diverse services as dental, drugs, home health, and vision care was the next largest single category in both years, and was higher in 1960 (31 cents) than in 1994 (24 cents). Physician services took 19 cents of the health expenditure dollar in 1960 and a very similar amount, 20 cents, in 1994. Nursing home care is one category that has doubled, taking only 4 cents of the

Figure 2-2a *The Nation's Health Dollar: 1960*

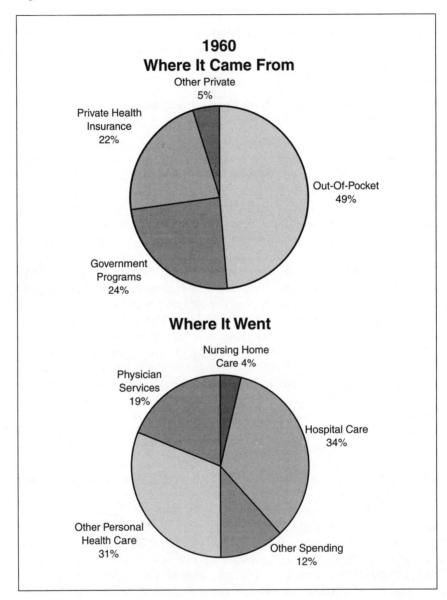

1960
Where It Came From

Other Private
5%

Private Health
Insurance
22%

Out-Of-Pocket
49%

Government
Programs
24%

Where It Went

Nursing Home
Care 4%

Physician
Services
19%

Hospital Care
34%

Other Personal
Health Care
31%

Other Spending
12%

SOURCE: Health Care Financing Administration, Office of the Actuary: Data from the Office of National Cost Estimates

NOTES: *Other Private* includes industrial in-plant health services, non-patient. revenues, and privately financed construction. *Other Personal Health Care* includes dental and other professional services, home health care, drugs and other non-durable medical products, and vision products and other durable medical products. *Other Spending* covers program administration and the net cost of private health insurance, government public health, and research and construction.

Figure 2-2b *The Nation's Health Dollar: 1994*

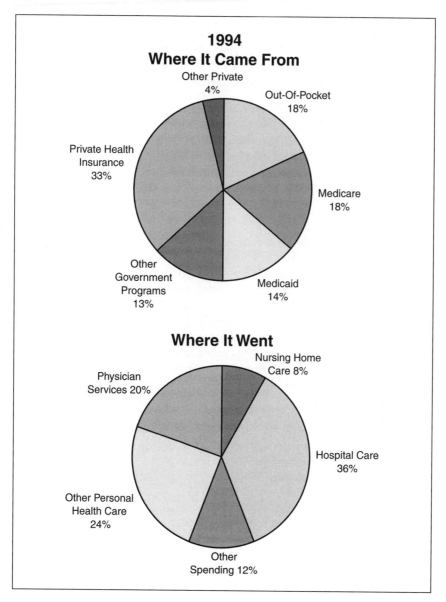

SOURCE: Health Care Financing Administration, Office of the Actuary: Data from the Office of National Cost Estimates

NOTES: *Other Private* includes industrial in-plant health services, non-patient revenues, and privately financed construction. *Other Personal Health Care* includes dental and other professional services, home health care, drugs and other non-durable medical products, and vision products and other durable medical products. *Other Spending* covers program administration and the net cost of private health insurance, government public health, and research and construction.

health care dollar in 1960 and 8 cents in 1994 (Levit et al., 1991b; Levit et al., 1996b; Office of National Cost Estimates, 1990).

Why are different types of health care expenditures increasing at varying rates? In the last 34 years, spending for hospital care grew most rapidly in the 1960s and 1970s. From 1966 to 1983, the average annual rate of growth in hospital revenues was 14 percent. In 1984, after the implementation of the DRG system for paying for hospital care delivered to Medicare recipients, the annual rate of growth in hospital care was cut in half to 7 percent, demonstrating that hospital cost containment programs are somewhat effective. Hospital revenues began to increase again in the late 1980s, increasing 10.1 percent from 1989 to 1990. From 1990 to 1994, rates of growth decelerated again, increasing only 4.4 percent in 1994 (Levit et al., 1991a; Levit et al., 1996b). Related to the decline in the rate of growth in expenditures for hospital care, admissions per capita have also been declining since the early 1980s, although in the last few years there have been almost no changes in admissions per population.

Most hospital care today is financed by insurance or government programs. One shift in the source of hospital revenues is that public funds and insurance together are paying more of the costs of hospital care, while the share of hospital care coming from out-of-pocket revenues has decreased from almost 21 percent in 1960 to 5 percent in 1990, and only 2.9 percent in 1994 (Levit et al., 1991b; Levit et al., 1996b). In fact, out-of-pocket payments for total health expenditures have decreased from 50 percent of national health expenditures in 1960 to 20 percent in 1990. The role of government and third-party payers has increased. Physician expenditures increased more rapidly in the decade of the 80s than did hospital care. Increases were more modest in the last few years, with growth of only 3.7 percent in 1993 and 4.6 percent in 1994. More of this area of expenditure is now covered by insurance or government, with a little less than 20 percent of physician services now being paid out of pocket versus 62 percent in 1960.

Most other areas of health expenditures are less well covered by insurance or government. In dental care, for example, almost half of all expenditures are still out of pocket. This is also true for prescription drug expenditures, medical supplies, durable medical equipment, and over-the-counter medications, although there is some variation. About 42 percent of prescription drug costs is paid out of pocket, whereas about 60 percent of durable products costs is paid for from out-of-pocket revenues, and almost all over-the-counter medications are paid for from out-of-pocket revenues. Vision products such as eyeglasses and contact lenses are the most important type of durable medical equipment (Levit et al., 1991b; Levit et al., 1996b).

The most rapidly growing category of health care expenditures is for home health care. This category has grown particularly rapidly since 1988. In that year, Medicare clarified and expanded its home health care coverage.

Public sources pay for almost three-quarters of all home health care, with over half of that paid by Medicare (Levit et al., 1991b).

The 1990s have been a period of changes in health expenditure patterns. Slow growth in personal health care use and intensity per person from 1992 to 1994 may indicate that insurer incentives have had some impact on controlling utilization. Hospital utilization rates per capita for the population under 65 have declined somewhat, as has length of stay. Some categories of spending, in contrast, have had double-digit rates of increase. The category of home health care services increased 22.5 percent from 1992 to 1993 and 13.8 percent from 1993 to 1994 (Levit et al., 1996b).

Personal health care expenditures account for about 90 percent of all national health expenditures, while supplies, research funds, and construction of medical care facilities account for the rest of expenditures (Levit et al., 1991b). Personal health expenses have been increasing at rates higher than the cost of living over the last 34 years, but have slowed more recently.

Why were the costs of health care increasing so dramatically in the United States? Why have they slowed in the past few years? The rates of growth in the 30-year period from 1960 to 1990 have exceeded both the general inflation rate and rates explainable by simple population growth alone. Obviously the increase in the proportion of the population that is elderly is one factor. In general, there has been an increase in the rate of use of services per capita and in the intensity of services provided (Gibson and Waldo, 1981; Levit et al., 1991b).

The implementation of Medicare and Medicaid did increase access for certain groups, and thus raised total expenditures. The biggest jump in health expenditures when viewed as a percentage of the total economy was in the late 1960s. Medicare, operating similarly to the overall Social Security system, provides federally sponsored health insurance to persons 65 years of age and over. The program also provides insurance to people with disabilities or the chronic disorder of end-stage renal disease (kidney failure). Medicaid operates as part of the patchwork blanket of state and federal welfare programs. Under Medicaid, federal and state governments jointly pay for hospital, physician, and additional services for eligible indigents. Given the welfare reform legislation enacted in 1996, states have greater flexibility in setting welfare policy and will limit the length of time that people can remain on the joint federal/state welfare programs. This may create some changes in the overall expenditures from the Medicaid program as these changes are gradually implemented in various states. Some protections have been retained to cover children, however, and it is too soon for any data to have been collected that might indicate the impact of welfare reform on Medicaid expenditures.

Changes in patterns by the different major types of payers have been under way in the past few years. Up until 1994, both Medicare and private health insurance encountered rapid benefit payment increases, about 13.7

percent for Medicare from 1969 to 1993 and 13.4 percent for private health insurance. In 1994, these growth patterns diverged, and spending for benefits for Medicare increased 11.8 percent while those for private health insurance increased only 4 percent (Levit, Lazerby, and Sivarajan, 1996a).

Additional factors that have contributed to increased costs are favorable attitudes toward the use of new medical technology and increased availability of health insurance (Kronenfeld and Whicker, 1984). Because more people have coverage for health insurance, they are more likely to seek out care. In addition, in the past, some physicians and hospitals provided charity care to those without insurance, and the cost of that care did not go into national expenditure figures.

One explanation for the difference in aggregate Medicare growth and private insurance growth is due to enrollment trends. The number of aged and disabled has been increasing over past decades. From 1969 to 1991, the increases averaged 2.5 percent annually. Since 1991, the annual increase has been 1.9 percent. In contrast, growth in enrollment in private health insurance has been 0.7 percent annually from 1969 to 1990 and 0.3 percent annually since 1991 (Levit et al., 1996a). Comparison between insurance sources is complicated because coverages of services and health care areas differ. More home health and nursing home services are covered by Medicare, and more prescription costs and dental care by private health insurance.

Technology can raise total health expenditures by creating types of services that did not even exist in the past. Costs go up particularly in the case of half-way technology, where medicine is able to help control a disease but not cure it (Fuchs, 1974). One of the best examples of the interaction between new technology and coverage for care has occurred in the treatment of kidney disease. Before the development of kidney dialysis, patients whose kidneys no longer functioned died in a short period of time. Dialysis machines are able to circulate the patient's blood through an artificial kidney located outside the body, removing toxic wastes and excess fluids. A typical regimen of therapy would last for 3 to 6 hours at a time, often three times a week. Since 1973, patients with this disease have been eligible for Medicare coverage. The annual cost of this treatment to the federal government is over $2 billion, for a disease affecting 70,000 patients (Kutner, 1982; Kutner, 1990; Plough, 1986). Technology can also reduce costs, at least the costs of a specific episode of care. A good example of this is the development of new technology that has made the removal of cataracts a quick, safe outpatient procedure over the last ten years, as compared to a two-week inpatient stay in the 1960s that was fraught with danger of loss of eyesight if a patient moved his or her head. Although the cost for the specific procedure has decreased greatly, this type of surgery has become the leading surgical expenditure for the Medicare program due to the success of the surgery and the aging of the population.

Controlling the Costs for the Government

While rising costs have been one of the major concerns of health policy experts in the 1980s and part of the 1990s, the review of expenditures for health care indicates that concern about rising costs, while it still exists, may be partially abating. Growth in health care costs has slowed so far in the 1990s (Levit et al., 1996b; Cowan et al., 1996; Service, 1995). A major concern in overall health care costs is that much of the savings has come from the shifting of people from more expensive indemnity health insurance plans into less expensive managed care plans (Service, 1995). Therefore, this may be only a one-time cost reduction. And even if this method of holding down overall health care costs works, the impact on government, both federal and state, is somewhat different. The federal government has continued to pay an ever-increasing share of the total health care bill, and issues about holding down costs both for Medicare (all federal funds) and Medicaid (joint federal and state funds) are still of major concern. Many of the newer pieces of federal legislation designed to deal with cost concerns will be discussed in more detail in later chapters.

One of the major pushes behind failed efforts at health care reform was to place controls on the growth of the Medicaid program and the attendant increase in health care costs for state governments. It is important to appreciate the impact that rising medical care costs have had on state budgets. In addition, problems in paying for Medicaid are related to issues of rising health care costs and uncovered health care costs (Fraser, Narcross, and Kralovec, 1991). Controversy abounds about Medicaid—because of rapidly increasing costs, periodic issues about quality of care, and its overall impact on state budgets and thus on state needs for tax and revenue increases, as well as on private insurance in the state.

How does Medicaid actually work? Coverage for the nation's poor is largely the responsibility of the Medicaid program, a joint federal-state entitlement program administered by states under broad federal guidelines. While many poor individuals are not covered by Medicaid, even the numbers currently covered (about 26 million people) are a major cost to state budgets. The federal government pays an average of 55 percent of the costs, a share that ranges from 50 percent to 80 percent depending upon a state's per capita income (Pepper Commission, 1990). States set their own criteria for eligibility—typically in line with the state's eligibility for Aid to Families of Dependent Children (AFDC) and extent of services—within federal guidelines. Thus a family of three in California in 1990 was eligible for Medicaid with a monthly income of $934, 106 percent of the federal poverty level that year, while the same family in Alabama would be eligible for Medicaid only if its income was $118 or less per month.

Over the past several years, Congress has mandated coverage up to higher income levels for some groups. The major focus of expansion since

1984 has been coverage for pregnant women and young children. The Omnibus Budget and Reconciliation Act (OBRA) of 1989 mandated that, beginning in April 1990, states had to cover pregnant women and children under age six with family incomes up to 133 percent of the federal poverty level. In addition, Congress mandated in 1988 that states had to continue Medicaid coverage for a year for beneficiaries who lose their eligibility for the program as their incomes increase. Both of these are worthwhile extensions from the perspective of access to care and improving health indicators. However, in many states, particularly those with less generous initial Medicaid coverage, the most rapidly increasing category of state expenditure has been the state match for the Medicaid program. A major concern in states has been the growth of what are called "entitlement" programs, typically joint federal-state programs where states do not control the numbers of people who become eligible but must come up with dollars to meet their share of the expense. In addition to Medicaid, AFDC and unemployment insurance operate similarly (although modified somewhat for AFDC with the reforms enacted in 1996). For Medicaid, however, the mandates have increased the costs of the program to states by expanding eligibility at the same time that costs of the actual medical care services have been increasing faster than general inflation and tax revenues. In many states, one of the largest single budget items is the Medicaid program, which then has become a major controversy as a result.

One way the programs have controlled total costs in the states is to hold down increases for specific categories, such as doctor's fees and hospital costs. In the last few years, state governments have responded to rising Medicaid spending by utilizing waiver programs to enroll more and more recipients into managed care health plans (Cowan et al., 1996). Thus the impact of Medicaid shortfalls reverberates throughout the entire health care system. Few health policy experts are naive enough to believe that health care costs are no longer a concern. In a political era in which the citizenry is interested in having no new taxes and in deficit reduction, the expenditures required for health care are a major concern—even if the rate of rising costs in health care has been slowing somewhat—and these issues will be part of any reexamination of health care reform and the role of government, both federal and state.

INDIVIDUAL AND INSTITUTIONAL PROVIDERS OF CARE

A major part of the health care delivery system in the United States is providers of care, whether we mean physicians; nurses, technicians, and aides; or institutional providers of care such as hospitals, ambulatory surgery centers, or nursing homes. In the past, both individual and institutional providers of care in the United States have been independent facets of the health care delivery system, with the role of the federal government limited to some training or research grants. (The details of the federal role in legislation, both in building the health care infrastructure and in more directly providing health care services, are covered in Chapter 4.) This section will review some basics about who individual and institutional providers are, how they have developed over time, how they have arrived at their current situations, and how providers currently link to both the dispersed and regionalist models of care found in the United States.

Different Types of Health Personnel

The number of different types of health care professionals and the numbers of people employed in the health care system have increased dramatically in the twentieth century. In 1910, only 1.3 percent of all employed people were in the health care sector. By 1950, this figure had almost doubled to 2.5 percent, and it doubled again in the next 30 years, up to 5.2 percent by 1980 (Moscovice, 1988). Currently, the health care industry is the largest single employer of all the industries monitored by the Department of Labor, its growth outpacing overall employment in the economy and total population growth. Issues about changes in health personnel policy and the role of the federal government in such changes are important in terms of both the responsibility of the health care industry for adequate delivery of health care and also for its role in the overall economy as a major employer.

Not only have the numbers of people employed in health care increased, but the types of jobs have changed and the numbers of different categories of health care workers have increased. Physicians, registered nurses, pharmacists, and dentists were the major categories of health care providers in 1910. Over the years, new groups have been added—optometrists, podiatrists, and physical therapists—with fairly high levels of specialized training. In addition, many new categories have been created, especially in the last thirty years, such as physicians' assistants, dental hygienists, laboratory technicians, practical nurses, nursing aides, home health aides, medical records personnel, respiratory therapists, and many other categories of allied health and support service personnel. There are now over 700 different job categories in the health industry.

Actually, it is the newer categories of health care providers whose numbers have increased the most. The traditional health care occupations of physicians, dentists, pharmacists, and optometrists have experienced dramatic declines in their relative proportion to all health care personnel, although the absolute numbers have increased in the last 30 years. Physicians comprised 30 percent of all persons in health care occupations in 1910, but only 9 percent by 1989 (Mick and Moscovice, 1993). Dentists have declined from 8 to 2 percent in the same time period, and pharmacists from 11 to 3 percent. Over two-thirds of all personnel now employed in health care are in nontraditional allied health or support service positions (Mick and Moscovice, 1993). One reason for this is the growth in technological innovation in the health care system in the last 30 years. As new types of machinery become available, often new allied health positions are created to specialize in the resultant new area of medicine and technology.

One traditional health care occupation, registered nursing, has continued to grow in large numbers. Registered nurses currently represent the largest single group of licensed health care personnel in the United States. Given the group's size and importance, specific policy issues such as what constitutes adequate staffing and what types of nurses will be needed in the health care system of the future. Nursing, an occupation in a state of flux, often confuses the public. The old image is that of women and caring, a field that provides a good temporary career for women until they marry and an appropriate feminine role for those who do not (Reverby, 1990). Nurses in the past provided a cheap labor pool for hospitals, and much of the care was provided by student nurses in training. During the Depression of the 1930s, the market for private-duty nurses disappeared and hospitals began to hire their own graduates at fairly low wages. The training for nurses, and even the employment practices, were exploitative and paternalistic; it was assumed that the hospital could control most of the life of the student nurse and even the registered nurse (RN) (Reverby, 1990, Weitz, 1996). Since the end of World War II, nurses have been committed to increasing their autonomy and improving both the conditions under which they work and their overall status within the health care field. However, the new image is unclear—at times that of overly technical, career-oriented professionals and at other times that of submissive women overworked and under the direction of doctors and administrators. One fact has changed little: Nurses are overwhelmingly women (over 95 percent).

One point of confusion is the multiple levels of nurses, particularly in hospital settings. The RN usually has a two- or four-year college degree, the most advanced training, and can perform a wide variety of tasks. This may include coordinating the care of patients in the hospital under the orders of a physician. Licensed practical or vocational nurses (LPNs) typically have a year of training and perform a variety of tasks under the nominal supervision of RNs. Nurses' aides generally have on-the-job training and perform the menial tasks of patient care, many of which involve personal hygiene. Within hospitals, the growth of reengineering and restructuring is changing both the roles of RNs and the use of other types of health personnel. Hospitals are moving away from employing as many LPNs or nurses' aides and also specialists within the various technology-oriented areas (such as laboratory technicians, respiratory therapists and phlebotomists). These personnel are being replaced by internally trained health care aides who can perform a variety of tasks, as long as the laws in that specific state do not require specific licensed personnel for those tasks. These types of changes in the care delivery model within the hospital often leave the RN with even more tasks to perform, although they may also increase the amount of management responsibility given the RN and, if implemented as part of a patient-focused care push, should increase the contact of the RN with the patient (Moffitt, Daly, Tracey, Galloway, and Tintsman, 1995).

Stratification within Health Care Professions

Many analysts of the health labor force agree on the dominant role of physicians, at least they did in the past (Aries and Kennedy, 1990; Freidson, 1970; Freidson, 1987; Starr, 1982). The medical profession and occupations related to it have undergone enormous changes in the past 20 to 30 years. Many believe the role of the physician is changing and that physicians' dominance over other health occupations is decreasing over time (McKinlay and Stoeckle, 1989). Other analysts have argued that the power relationship between doctors and patients is also changing, leading to a deprofessionalization among physicians (Haug, 1976; Haug, 1988). Recently, experts have argued that the growth of HMOs (health maintenance organizations) and managed care groups has changed the power relationship between physicians and nonmedical administrators and led to the challenge of the professional and clinical judgment of physicians. This process has been called proletarianization and corporatization by sociologists and is described as a shift in managerial roles by health administration experts (Kaluzny and Shortell, 1997).

What are other factors changing the role of dominance of physicians? The financing of health care has been viewed by some as an important factor (Aries and Kennedy, 1990), linked to the growth in HMOs and managed care. Also, even though the rise in health care costs has slowed in the last few years, the past experience of rapidly rising health care costs has raised public concern about physicians' salaries. While costs of physician care are only one element of rising costs, it is often a visible element.

Physicians traditionally have played the dominant role in the health care occupations, setting the terms and conditions of work for all the others. They have been the group that earned the most, and either directly or indirectly hired many of the other workers. Physicians traditionally have dominated the determination of licensure and certification requirements and have overseen exams for many of the technical health occupations. Freidson has characterized physicians as being "technically autonomous," that is, being able to set their own conditions of work (Freidson, 1970). Physicians have also had the right to limit and evaluate the performance of most other health care workers. The profession of medicine is undergoing challenges to its position now, which is part of a reorganization of the delivery of health care in the United States—and perhaps part of a period in American history in which there is generally greater suspicion of formal authority and more questioning of "professional" experts of any type. On the other hand, physicians still rank at the top of a hierarchy of health care occupations. Other types of health care professionals mostly do work that helps physicians to function, they do not engage directly in the critical tasks of diagnosis of the problem or prescription of care (with the exception of some of the nurse practitioner roles now emerging), and they earn far less, with more limited opportunities for advancement in earnings or job diversity.

The growth of the consumer movement has resulted in a challenge to physicians' autonomy (Haug, 1976). The trust by consumers in the advice of all types of professionals is declining, partially because the modern consumer is better educated. He or she is more likely to comprehend medical subjects, thus decreasing the knowledge gap between consumers and health care providers.

The passage of the Medicare and Medicaid legislation in 1965 committed vast amounts of federal funds into the health care system, but it also ultimately made the costs of health care more visible. At the same time that improved access was increasing total dollars in the health care system and improved technology was raising total costs, labor costs within the health care sector became an issue. At one time, the major providers in health care were physicians who operated as small private businesses and nurses who were poorly paid, both because of the origins of nursing as a charitable enterprise and because it was a female-dominated field, and female fields have traditionally paid more poorly within the American economy (Reverby, 1990). However, nursing salaries have increased in the last 30 years, as have salaries of other less trained hospital workers. For many of these health care workers, increases in the minimum wage and unionization movements have helped in obtaining increases in pay. Because 60 percent of hospital costs are attributed to labor inputs, labor costs are the most likely source of savings in that sector of the health care system in the future (Aries and Kennedy, 1990). The role that government at any level, including the federal government, should play in future decisions about various types of health care personnel, and relative power between groups, is not an easily resolved issue.

Medicine and the Appropriate Supply of Physicians

The issue of having an appropriate number of physicians in practice has long been a major concern in the United States. Several difficulties occur in achieving these objectives. The first is determining what is the appropriate number of physicians. The second is determining what supply trends really are, how rapidly they are changing or may change, and how these link to changing roles of physicians within the health care delivery system. The number of physicians in the United States has increased rapidly in the last two decades, with an 84 percent increase in the supply of physicians between 1970 and 1990. Two different trends account for the higher numbers—an increase in the number of graduates from medical schools since 1965 and substantial immigration of foreign physicians into the United States. Before 1970, the general belief was that the United States had too few physicians. Historically, students graduating from U.S. medical schools had filled only two-thirds to three-quarters of all the residencies available in U.S. hospitals. Thus in the 1960s and 1970s, there were large new federal outlays for training of medical students and construction of new medical schools, to increase the supply of physicians. These policies began to take effect, and numbers increased, as illustrated in Table 2-1, which shows the changes in the supply of physicians from 1970 to 1990.

Beginning in 1980, the Graduate Medical Education National Advisory Committee (GMENAC) warned of a surplus of 70,000 physicians by 1990 (GMENAC, 1980). This was a controversial conclusion at the time, with many experts arguing that it underestimated the changing patterns of medical school enrollment and preferences for less than excessive hours of work. Also, critiques pointed to a lack of attention to short supply in certain fields, especially primary care fields such as family practice, and inadequate staffing in certain parts of the country, particularly rural areas (Barnett and Midling, 1989). The number of female medical students was increasing, and evidence was growing that both young female and male physicians desired to work fewer hours than the 60 to 80 hour workweeks typical of many older physicians. Depending upon the assumptions of how many hours the typical physician of the future will work, the estimates of physician supply vary greatly.

In general, these estimates of oversupply did not turn out to be true for 1990. For whatever reasons, from 1987 through 1990 the number of applicants to U.S. medical schools dropped, and this caused a particular drop in

Table 2-1 *Number of Active Physicians: 1970, 1980, 1990*

Health Occupation	1970		1980		1990[a]	
	Number	Personnel per 100,000 Population	Number	Personnel per 100,000 Population	Number	Personnel per 100,000 Population
Physicians	326,200	156.0	457,500	197.0	601,060	240.0
MDs	314,200	150.0	440,400	189.5	543,310	228.9
DOs	12,000	6.0	17,100	7.5	27,570	11.1

[a] Estimated data.

SOURCES: *Fourth report to the President and Congress on the status of health personnel in the United States* (DHHS Publication No. [HRS]-P-0084.4) (1984 May). Washington, DC: U.S. Government Printing Office; *Seventh report to the President and Congress on the status of health personnel in the United States* (DHHS Publication No. [HRS]-P-OD-90-1) (1990 March). Washington, DC: U.S. Government Printing Office.

the number of potential residents in internal medicine, family practice, and, to a lesser extent, pediatrics (Colwill, 1992). In 1991, 19 percent fewer U.S. medical school graduates entered residencies in these specialties than in 1986. In addition, actual applications to medical schools declined. Controversy exists as to why these declines have occurred. One consideration was that the primary care incomes were not keeping up with specialty incomes and that the declining applications were a response (Colwell, 1992; Petersdorf, 1992). A different, although related, explanation is that specialists receive more professional and general respect and prestige, which explains the lessening of interest in generalist care (Petersdorf, 1992). Medical school applications are rising again in the 1990s, even though growing numbers of physicians (38 percent in a recent study) now say they would not recommend medicine as a career choice to a high school or college student (Harvey and Shubat, 1990). There is also evidence now that numbers of medical students interested in primary care fields are growing again, and that more students are choosing these fields—whether as a response to higher reimbursements in the modified physician payment approaches of the government, to higher starting salaries for generalists with HMOs resulting from the growth of managed care, or to the growing perception of an oversupply of most specialists (Schroeder, 1996) is unclear.

Nursing and Supply of Personnel

Compared to the staffing for medicine, nursing has had a more cyclical supply picture. At some points in the last thirty years there has been an oversupply, while in other years there has been a shortage (Moccia, 1990; Moscovice, 1988; Newschaffer and Schoenman, 1990). While there has been a perception of cyclical nursing shortages in the past, characterized by some improvements in salary and additional recruits into the field, stability in numbers or an oversupply, stagnation of salaries, and then gradual perceptions of a renewed shortage, the situation for the last five years appears to have shifted. There were clear shortages in 1979–80 and 1986–88 relative to number of positions to be filled, even if the absolute numbers of nurses available were high (Newschaffer and Schoenman, 1990). By 1985, there were more nurses (both RNs and LPNs) than ever before, a higher labor force participation rate among RNs than in any other period (over 80 percent), and more nurses working in hospitals than ever in recent history (over 68 percent), yet there was a perception of a shortage—particularly in the hospital sector (Moccia, 1990). One argument has been that nurses do not remain in the same positions for long, creating the impression of continued shortages.

A major question is whether there continues to be a shortage, one that will become worse in future years as more and more technology leads to the need for more nurses, while few women (and even fewer men) enroll in nursing programs. Alternatively, are we coming out of another cycle and are numbers of new entrants into nursing again increasing? Some argue that nursing enrollments are up (Mayer, 1991; Newschaffer and Schoenman, 1990; "Nursing School Enrollments Up," 1992). Others argue that the availability of alternative careers for women—especially alternative careers within medicine—will lead to a continued problem of nursing shortages (Delevan and Koff, 1990). In the last four years, the increased reengineering and restructuring of hospitals, the closing of some and merging of others into unified systems, have led to reductions in the numbers of RNs employed in many cities in the United States. While there is not currently an oversupply, many experts believe that nursing positions will become more difficult to locate, and that more jobs will require advanced skills (as nurse practitioners) or the willingness to function in a changed health care setting as hospitals are reorganized to produce care more efficiently.

Settings of Care

Thus far, this chapter has reviewed topics related to the costs of care, and the history of and current issues concerning providers of health care services. Much of the rest of this section will focus upon similar background data and current issues having to do with where care is provided (sites) rather than who provides it. The review will explore, in turn, ambulatory or outpatient care, HMOs, hospital-based care, and systems of care.

Ambulatory Care, Managed Care and HMOs

One of the major growth areas in health care today and over the last 10 to 15 years is ambulatory care. More and more services, such as outpatient surgery and advanced types of diagnostic procedures, are being provided in that setting. While in the recent past, ambulatory care was delivered in doctors' offices or in a few outpatient settings such as hospital clinics, at the turn of the century, much ambulatory care was provided in the patient's own home, with the physician carrying the tools and supplies needed to provide care in that far less technological era. Today, the sites of such care are more varied and can include special facilities for outpatient surgeries, emergency care and walk-in clinics, and group care settings such as health maintenance organizations (HMOs), in addition to the more traditional doctor's office.

Health maintenance organizations typically combine the provision of health care services with an insurance function. The older type of HMO would be an organization such as Kaiser that provides care in group settings, may run its own hospitals, and is the insurance plan in that it is the group to which premiums are paid. Such plans usually cover almost all health care services, with minimal fees at the time a patient receives care—such as a $5 or $10 co-payment for a doctor visit or a prescription. Newer types of provisions include IPAs (individual practice associations), in which the insurance plan contracts with a number of different providers to give care—often at their own office locations. One idea behind such plans is to create an incentive to keep the patient well (hence the name *health maintenance* organization) by having the plan financially at risk for most of care. This placement of risk on the plan or the group of doctors rather than the patient should create greater emphasis on preventive care, on finding problems at an early stage, and treating them when they are smaller. Recent studies have found that HMOs provide a good quality of care, equaling or exceeding that found in traditional health insurance arrangements (Luft, 1981). One study found that HMO clients receive between 25 and 50 percent fewer surgical operations than do patients in fee-for-service programs, but with no difference in health outcomes (Leape, 1992).

Although the older HMOs such as Kaiser are nonprofit, much of the growth in the last 20 years has been through for-profit HMOs (Kronenfeld and Whicker, 1990). Now a term used increasingly is *managed care,* which is a generic term that encompasses a variety of forms of prepaid and managed fee-for-service health care (Williams and Torrens, 1993b). The number of HMOs more than doubled from 1980 to 1990, and has continued increasing during the 1990s. The most rapidly growing segment of the managed care market is the insurer-owned managed care plan (Hoy, Curtis, and Rice, 1991). In 1990, managed care plans comprised 25 percent of the market for members of the Health Insurance Association of America, up from only 1 percent in 1982 (Hoy et al., 1991). Nationwide, HMO enrollment in 1994 increased by 5.3 million people, to over 50 million Americans. This was an 11 percent increase in membership in one year, the largest single-year enrollment jump, and followed large increases of 7.3 percent and 9.2 percent in membership in 1992 and 1993 (Service, 1995).

One concern is what the future direction of growth may be and which companies are likely to be the major providers in the next 10 years. Large HMOs have bought smaller ones in record numbers in the last few years. For example, in June 1994, FHP International Corporation acquired another large California-based HMO to become the fifth largest HMO in the United States. In this kind of merger, one concern is what happens to patients and whether the moves are good for individuals—or only for the companies. In the last few years, many publicly traded HMOs have reported earnings growth of 25 percent or more (Service, 1995). Past history highlights some patient concerns: For example, in 1986 Maxicare had over 2 million members and was touted as the best-managed HMO in the industry. It filed for bankruptcy protection three years later (Christianson, Wholey, and Sanchez, 1991). On the other hand, some companies such as Cigna have been successful with both numbers of enrollees and profits.

Another concern is whether economic incentives may be uppermost and lead to undertreatment of medical conditions. Some of these concerns link to attitudes of the public. Over the last two years, consumer satisfaction with HMOs has been slipping, with the proportion of HMO enrollees who report being satisfied having fallen slightly from 63.6 percent in 1994 to 59.3 percent in 1996 (Jensen, 1996). In surveys of enrollees, satisfaction with quality of care and outcomes has decreased significantly in the past two years, partially because over a fourth of HMO enrollees have experienced problems in obtaining referrals to a specialist. Despite this decline, the rate of satisfaction of HMO enrollees exceeds that of those in fee-for-service and PPO (preferred provider organization) plans.

A number of health reform plans envision a model of competing HMOs as one way to reorganize the health care system to provide more comprehensive care to most patients and yet control costs. In some ways, this model was part of the failed Clinton health care reform plan in his first term. While HMOs are growing rapidly, the experience to date varies in different sectors of the country. HMOs are most common in the western portions of the United States, in Minnesota, and in the areas around major population centers in the East and Northeast (Washington, DC, Boston, New York City); they are least common in the Southeast and rural portions of the West and Midwest. Experience with managed care is growing in many parts of the country, for example through the expansion of managed care into the Medicare and Medicaid programs. The elderly are most likely to enroll in Medicare HMOs in the same areas of the country in which general HMO enrollment is high. For Medicaid, more and more states are expanding on the model of a managed care Medicaid program first started as a statewide program in Arizona in the mid-1980s. Recently, Tennessee has converted the entire state Medicaid program to a managed care model, even though overall HMO market penetration in the state at the time was only 6 percent (Service, 1995). Thus, in various ways, both through the growth of the use of HMOs in the workplace and the expansion of HMOs in Medicare and Medicaid, more and more people are receiving ambulatory care in this type of arrangement.

Hospital History and Current Structure

Hospitals have played an important role in the delivery of health care services in the United States for at least the past 60 years, and perhaps as far back as 1900. Up to now, the modern hospital, especially in the post–World War II era, has been the key resource and organizational hub of the U.S. health care system. It has been central to delivery of patient care, training of personnel, and conduct and dissemination of health-related research (Haglund and Dowling, 1984). Hospitals are important both in the total amount of health care delivered and as a major employment sector. They are the second- or third-largest industry in the United States in terms of numbers of people employed, and they employ about three-quarters of all the health care workers. Whether hospitals will remain the key resource and organizational hub of the health care system is one of the major policy questions concerning the organization and structure of the health care delivery system in the twenty-first century.

The history of hospitals is long, but not in the versions we think of today (Rosenberg, 1987; Stevens, 1989). The early origins of the hospital trace back to almshouses—poorhouses and workhouses established by city and county government—that evolved into specialized institution to care for the sick poor (Rosenberg, 1987). In the late 1700s and early 1800s, some voluntary hospitals began to emerge, often at the urging of physicians who wanted places in which to practice surgery in the manner in which they had been taught in Europe. By the late 1800s, the growth of modern science, the development of the germ theory of disease, and, the control of infections through aseptic technique—as well as the application of anesthesia in surgery—all combined with more general societal trends of industrialization and urbanization to create a more important role for hospitals as the providers of care, not just to the poor but to a growing middle class and even to the wealthy (Rosenberg, 1987).

There have really been two traditions of hospital services in the United States, one the private sector—partially nonprofit and particularly so after World War II—and one the public sector (Kronenfeld and Whicker, 1990). Hospital care for the poor was concentrated in county or municipal hospitals until the introduction of the Medicaid program in 1965. The private sector consisted of voluntary hospitals including typical community hospitals, those affiliated with religious associations, and other types of nonprofit facilities (Stevens, 1989). At the turn of the century, most for-profit hospitals were run by physicians and were often set up in smaller and rural communities to provide a place in which to practice for an individual doctor or a few doctors in town. Half of hospitals in the United States were for-profit in 1900. This proportion decreased over the course of the twentieth century, so that by 1970 only 13 percent of hospitals were for-profit (Kronenfeld and Whicker, 1990).

How hospital care has been paid for since 1920 is very important in understanding the major policy issues today. Up until World War II, most hospital care for middle-class people was paid for through savings. The Depression caused major problems for hospital incomes, both because people could not pay for care and because charitable donations for care of the poor were down. The financial solvency of many hospitals was threatened, leading to the idea of voluntary group hospitalization plans, especially through Blue Cross (Haglund and Dowling, 1993; Stevens, 1989). Private insurance for hospital care grew rapidly, so that by 1965 most of the working population had third-party insurance to cover hospital stays. With the introduction of Medicare for the elderly and Medicaid for the poor in 1965, important groups of people who did not previously have money or insurance to pay for care received other options.

The growth of private insurance and the two governmental programs initially provided enormous revenues for hospitals in the United States. The public plans and private insurance together ensured the financial stability of hospitals and increased the demand for their services. Because many people had coverage for hospital care but not outpatient care in the 1960s, demand for hospital care was quite high, even for services that probably could have been performed outside the hospital. One study examining hospital admissions from 1974 to 1982 found that 23 percent of admissions studied were inappropriate, and 17 percent could have been avoided through the use of outpatient surgery (Siu, Sonnenberg, Manning, Goldberg, Blumfield, Newhouse, and Brooke, 1986).

Hospitals, then, enjoyed a period of growth and prosperity. Actual numbers of hospitals declined slightly from 1971 to 1990, however, going from 7,678 in 1971 to 6,595 in 1990 (*Hospital Statistics*, 1991; National Center for Health Statistics, 1971). Much of this decline was due to a decrease in the number of governmental hospitals, while the numbers of nonprofit hospitals declined slightly and the numbers of for-profit hospitals actually increased from 1971 to 1990. One other important trend in this time period was the decline in hospitals with a smaller number of beds, as some consolidation began to occur and as smaller, rural hospitals with few beds were replaced by more centrally located facilities in larger population centers near rural areas.

The method of reimbursement used by most private insurers and initially by Medicare—cost-based reimbursement—led to high costs. In that system, hospitals simply passed along all the costs of providing services directly to the third-party payor. There was no incentive for the hospital to contain costs, leading to rapidly rising expenses in the late 1960s and 1970s. Rising hospital costs was a major factor leading to the passage, in 1982, of the diagnostic related groups (DRG) reimbursement system as part of the Tax Equity and Fiscal Responsibility Act of 1982. This converted the way Medicare paid for hospital care from a cost-based reimbursement system to a prospective per-case system based on the diagnosis of the patient, with over 460 different diagnosis-related payment categories. Instead of a hospital being able to charge a patient a set fee per day plus specific charges for supplies and other special facilities, the care of Medicare patients is now paid with one fee, set in advance, based on the expected average length of stay and services used. Many states now also reimburse the hospital stays of Medicaid patients by the same formula. Thus, for hospitals, whereas before they could almost be certain of breaking even or having excess revenues on the care of every patient except for charity cases or bad debts (where no one paid), they must now figure out how to provide care at the preset fees provided by Medicare (and in some states, Medicaid). Since elderly people use the most hospital care, this reimbursement change affects half or more of most hospital stays; how to break even has suddenly become a major issue for hospitals. Managing a hospital has shifted from being a situation in which a manager was almost sure to be successful to being one of trying to maximize the types of patients and revenue they represent, at any given time, while still keeping the hospital staff (and the community, in the case of nonprofit community facilities) reasonably satisfied.

There are often two or more ways of considering many issues. This is particularly true when we examine hospital care costs. Earlier in this chapter, we looked at costs from a perspective of the total society and the governmental sector. From that perspective, controlling the amount of dollars spent on hospital care is good. From the perspective of a hospital administrator, however, any decrease in dollars spent on health care raises questions of how hospitals of the future will pay their bills. The whole intent of the shift to DRG-based payment for hospital services for Medicare patients was to slow the rate of increase in government expenses for hospital care, both by holding down the costs of each specific hospitalization and possibly also by lowering the numbers of admissions, since new peer review organizations were also set up to monitor inpatient care for appropriateness of treatment. Most experts now agree that the changes in Medicare did slow spending for hospital inpatient care significantly (Christianson et al., 1991). Also, admission rates declined from 1983 through 1987, and rates in 1989 for people 65 and over were still only 85 percent of rates in 1983 (Christianson et al., 1991). Overall occupancy rates have also declined, and there has been a wave of hospital closures, mostly in inner city and rural locations.

It may be that hospitals are losing their dominance over health care. More and more procedures and surgery are now performed in outpatient settings. Third-party payers, such as insurance companies, are able to dictate terms of treatment. More after-hospital care is now being provided in patients' homes and long-term care facilities, as a way to hold down costs and maximize the revenues from DRG-based payments by shifting the patient from the hospital to other care settings. In any event, there is now great controversy and ambiguity over the future role of hospitals. Those in the United States have long represented the values of science and, as a result, have carried important cultural weight. They have also represented charity and caring, particularly in the nonprofit sector, both religiously and nonreligiously based. Earlier in the century they also represented forces for social order. All of these values are shifting, with a greater emphasis on hospitals as businesses. Moreover, with more and more advanced care now occurring in other settings, will hospitals become only a collection of specialized workshops? Will the notion of the hospital extend beyond the walls of the institution to the application of medical care technology in a wide variety of service settings, with the hospital basically becoming the health care system? A major expert on hospitals, Stevens (1989), concludes that hospitals in the United States are in flux. She argues that we have a de facto national health system available through our hospitals, but are unwilling to recognize the fact and that "while the American hospital industry has major deficiencies as a public service, as a largely private industry it has been enormously successful" (Stevens, 1989, pp. 352–353).

A major trend of the 1990s has been the growth of multihospital systems. More than half of all the beds in U.S. hospitals today are part of a multihospital system that is made up of two or more acute-care facilities (Haglund and Dowling, 1993). A growing trend is that more and more of these systems are investor-owned. Today, the investor-owned systems are among the largest, often including over 20 hospitals, scattered across various geographic areas of the United States.The largest single hospital chain, Columbia/HCA Healthcare Corporation, had over 311 hospitals and 125 clinics in 37 states and two foreign countries in 1995 and was planning further expansion ("The State of Health Care in America," 1995).

Another trend among hospitals has been the building of strategic alliances (Zajac and D'Aunno, 1997). About 30 percent of the nation's hospitals are members of alliances, and there are 15 large alliances with over 1,600 members. Alliances can be formed among hospitals and physician groups, hospitals and HMOs, and groups of hospitals.

All of these trends are part of a reaction to a rapidly changing world of health services delivery, in which the methods of the past do not necessarily lead to success in the future. Some of the alliance formation of the early 1990s was in anticipation of expected government reform; this did not occur in a major way. The processes of consolidation, however, have not ceased. Health care experts currently see several different models of care and organizational relationships that could emerge, depending partially on government actions as well as on evolving social norms and expectations. Suggested options include an organized delivery system, community care networks, and greater growth of alliances (Kaluzny and Shortell, 1997). An organized delivery system is something like that described in Chapter 1 as a regionalist model, and which HMOs partially represent, but which would probably require major governmental action to become the overall way of care delivery in the United States. Community care networks advance the idea of including broad-based health and social services such as are typically associated with public health and public welfare departments, along with health care services, with the locus of control at the community level—and no part of the United States currently fits this model of care. Alliance formation continues to occur. All of these ideas link to the notion of broader frameworks for caring for individuals, the continuum of care.

A CONTINUUM OF CARE: PREVENTION, ACUTE, CHRONIC, AND LONG-TERM

As the U.S. health care system has been undergoing change over the last decade, one idea that was initially discussed as part of long-term care and is now receiving more discussion overall is the continuum of care (Bean and Waldron, 1995; Evashwick, 1993; Lumsdon, 1994; Porter-O'Grady, 1995). Long-term care is usually defined as the health, mental health, social, and residential services that are provided to temporarily or chronically disabled persons over an extended period of time with a goal of enabling them to function as independently as possible (Evashwick, 1993). In the past, the primary users of long-term care have been the elderly and other persons with chronic or long-term complex health problems that lead to functional disabilities. Since 1965, both the aging of the U.S. population and greater availability of access to health care on the part of the elderly and the disabled due to the Medicare and Medicaid programs have increased the use of long-term care services (Wallace, Abel, and Stefanowicz, 1996). As both these services and concern over the costs of nursing home care (the oldest type of long-term care services) have grown, discussion has shifted to talk about all the services individuals may need to manage their health. Over 80 different services have been identified as part of a complete continuum of care, including ambulatory care, home care, acute care, extended care, outreach services, wellness and health promotion services, and housing services.

The essence of a continuum is an integrated system of care. In the long-term care arena, growth of the notion of continuum has been associated with the development of case-management and the creation of a position who becomes responsible for helping to coordinate all the care of a patient (Lumsdon, 1994; Porter-O'Grady, 1995). Experts who have worked on creating a continuum of care for long-term care patients argue that the future of health care lies in harnessing the power of information and learning to track costs, providers, and sources of care and to connect them with clinical outcomes (Lumsdon, 1994). The future has also been linked with accountability, and with a focus on outcomes of care rather than a process of care (Porter-O'Grady, 1995). The notion is better developed within the long-term philosophy, and one lesson learned from that area is that if a continuum of care is to function as a system of care, rather than as a fragmented collection of services, integrating mechanisms are needed. Among the most important are 1) an internal organization that coordinates the operations of various systems, 2) a management information system that integrates clinical, utilization, and financial data and follows clients across settings, 3) a case-management/care-coordination program that works with clients to arrange services, and 4) a financing mechanism that enables pooling of funds across services.

If the new world of managed care becomes the major way of the future—whether through the independent workings of the health care marketplace, or because of a renewed emphasis on health care reform and attention paid to creation of a new model of care in the United States that is similar to the regionalized model of care (Grumbach and Bodenheimer, 1995)—organized delivery systems may be the method of the future (Shortell, Gillies, and Anderson, 1994). For these models to be complete and improve the health care of most Americans, as they move out of the long-term care arena and into all types of care across the total age-span, they will need to include both prevention of health care problems and concern about maintenance of health, not just concern about integration of services provided to individuals. Perhaps this new system will emerge through the private marketplace, or perhaps major government changes will cause a move toward a more integrated continuum of care or even create an overall organized system of health care delivery in the United States. As the system changes, its most salient features will also change.

This chapter has reviewed some of the most prominent aspects of the present U.S. health care system, and speculated a bit on where changes are currently leading. One major question is the role of government in the future shape of the U.S. health care system. Part Two will review the policy formation process in this country and then examine major types of federal health-related legislation. Part Three will review the attempts at major health care reform in the first term of the Clinton presidency. It will end with a discussion of the possibilities for the future of both the federal role in health care delivery and the organization of the U.S. health care delivery system.

Part II
The Federal Legislative Process and Its Outcome

3 HEALTH POLICY PROCESS AT THE NATIONAL LEVEL AND THE ROLE OF POLITICS

Health policy occupies an important place in the domestic policy agenda of the United States. In the last decade, one major effort at comprehensive health care reform has occurred as part of a public policy discussion (the failed Clinton health care reform plan proposed in the first two years of his first term of office), and more minor reforms of the health care system were passed eventually as part of a bipartisan effort near the end of the first Clinton term, a period during which the Republican party had recaptured the control of Congress (both Senate and House of Representatives) for the first time in half a century. Moreover, even though health issues were not a focal part of the discussion during the 1996 presidential election, there were 11 initiatives relating to health care on the ballots of six western states (the states most likely to have an initiative option as part of how state government functions) for the November 1996 election (Page, 1996).

While this book focuses upon federal health policy, federal and state policy interact in a number of issue areas, including health. Additionally, health policy is not a simple subject, and it is linked to and is similar to a number of other policy areas. A nation's health policy is part of its general overall social policy. As a result, health policy formulation is influenced by the variety and array of social and economic factors that impact social policy development. The nature and history of existing institutions, the general climate of opinion, ritualized methods for dealing with social conflict, attitudes and behavioral characteristics of key political actors, and the general goals and values of a society all play a role in the formulation of social policy (Fein, 1980; Kronenfeld and Whicker, 1984). The first section of this chapter will define both policy and health policy, and describe the forms of

health policies. The second section will discuss the basic political philosophies that are found in the United States and their link to the structure of
our governmental system—federalism—and how federalism impacts policy issues. The next section will describe a model of public policy making
for health, and discuss the processes of policy formulation, implementation, and modification. The last section will examine the changing role of
interest groups in the political process in the United States, and present
competing arguments explaining why it is difficult within the U.S. political
system to achieve major policy reforms in many areas, including the area of
health care reform.

DEFINITIONS AND FORMS OF HEALTH POLICY

Public policies are authoritative decisions made in the legislative, executive, or judicial branches of government intended to direct or influence the
actions, behaviors, or decisions of others (Longest, 1994). If a policy relates
to the pursuit of health, the employment of health care professionals, or the
receipt of health care services, it is a part of health care policy. Government
currently plays a major role in the United States in the planning, directing,
and financing of health care services, even though at an earlier time this
was far less true. Close to half of the nation's personal health expenditures
now are paid for with public funds, and most physicians and other health
care personnel are trained partially through federal funds that form a type
of indirect—if not direct—subsidy to the colleges and universities that they
attend. About 45 percent of the research and development funds in the
United States are provided by all units of government, with the bulk being
provided by the federal government, although this is a lower percentage
than ten years ago, when the proportion was over 50 percent. Despite the
current extensive impact of the federal government in many aspects of
health care delivery, health professions, and health research, these programs have evolved in a piecemeal fashion, and often in response to needs
unmet by the private sector or state or local government. While the direct
role of the federal government had been focussed on the increase in health
policy making from 1930 until 1980, at that point the Reagan administration tried to diminish significantly the federal role in domestic social policy, including health policy. From then to now, the country has had
continuing debates over whether programs should expand or contract and
whether states, or the federal government, or private industry and the
workings of the marketplace should play a more major role. Stated differently, we are in a period of questioning of government. Because of this, and
the failure of major health care reform in 1993–94, the direction in health
care in the last few years has been influenced more by nongovernmental
trends than was true in the period from 1965–85.

Despite this questioning, health policy decisions are made by government every day, whether at the national, state, or, occasionally, local level. Health policy includes a large body of decisions. Some are what we most often think of as laws—that is, pieces of legislation passed by Congress. Most of what we think of as major federal health care programs, such as Medicare, were passed initially as laws (in the case of Medicare, as Title XVIII to the Social Security Legislation and also known as PL 89-97, which created the Medicare program in the mid 1960s). Other policy decisions are found in the rules and regulations established by agencies in the executive branch in order to be able to operate government, since most pieces of legislation are relatively brief and lacking in the details needed for implementation as they leave Congress. Over the years, the amount of rules and regulations explaining how Medicare and its modifications work grew much larger in bulk and importance than the specific pieces of legislation themselves. Another way policies are made is by the judicial branch, in reviewing a case that relates to health issues. One important recent example was a decision in 1992 by a U.S. Department of Health and Human Services administrative law judge that a hospital had violated the Rehabilitation Act Amendments of 1974 (PL 93-516) when it had prohibited an HIV-positive staff pharmacist from preparing intravenous solutions. This decision has helped to protect the rights of health care workers who are HIV-positive to remain employed within the health care sector.

THE LINKAGES OF POLITICAL PHILOSOPHY AND FEDERALISM

As stated earlier, a nation's health policy is part of its general overall social policy and, as a result, health policy formulation is influenced by the variety and array of social and economic factors that impact broader policy development issues in the United States. The nature and history of existing institutions, the general climate of opinion, ritualized methods for dealing with social conflict, and general goals and values of a society all play a role in the formulation of such policy. Important aspects of American society that need to be understood to appreciate the policy process in the United States include the basic ideological orientation of the United States and the system of federalism and the historical circumstances that have produced and modified it over time.

Political Philosophy

An important overall factor in understanding the policy process in the United States is its basic ideological orientation. There are two aspects of this: the economic system of capitalism and the political orientation of classical liberalism (or perhaps, given the usage today of conservative and liberal as descriptors of sides of the political spectrum, individualism).

Classical liberalism or individualism emphasizes individuals as the basis and justification for the creation of government, and has been one basic ideological orientation of the United States since its founding. This approach was developed in Europe in the eighteenth century and transplanted to and nurtured in the United States. In order to protect against government imposing arbitrary choices upon citizens, government and governmental policies were seen as most effective if they remained small in scale, so that individuals could attain maximum choice. Most things affecting individual well-being, including responsibility for personal health care, were to be both the choice and the responsibility of the individual. Only in the twentieth century did liberals begin to see government as a counter to other powerful forces within society that impinged upon individual freedom. On the other hand, while the attitude toward the role of government shifted somewhat—to regard big government and government policies as a sometimes necessary evil to counter other forces, particularly economic—the supreme emphasis on the individual remained.

Strongly related to political liberalism is its economic philosophical twin: capitalism. Capitalism emphasizes the operation of a free-market economy and competition. Combined with this is a belief that overall society would be better off if each individual within it vigorously pursues his or her welfare to the greatest extent possible. Capitalism was also initially articulated in the eighteenth century, with the publication of Adam Smith's groundbreaking book, *The Wealth of Nations* in 1776, the year of the American Revolution. Its simultaneous birth with that of the United States as a country makes it understandable that capitalism would be adopted by the new nation (Macridis, 1983).

Capitalism represented a significant departure from the prevailing Christian philosophy, especially within Catholicism, that had generally dominated thinking up to that time. Christianity maintained that society was better off as a whole if each individual within it adhered to norms of self-denial and a lessening of concern about personal gain. By contrast, capitalist theory contended almost the reverse: that society was to be better off as a whole if each individual within it vigorously pursued his or her own welfare to the greatest extent possible. Capitalism, as well as some of the growing Protestant religions, glorified individual gain (Weber, 1958).

Capitalism operated through private markets in which individuals were free to choose jobs, investments, and consumption patterns. The driving force was competition, where no single unit of production controlled either the total quantity or price of a good or service. Government intervention, under capitalistic theory, was neutral at best and usually malevolent (Friedman, 1962). Only in the late 1800s and early 1900s was government intervention perceived as necessary to regulate and enforce competition in the private marketplace through antitrust legislation. At that point, government became a referee among powerful private corporations and wealthy industrialists trying to build financial empires.

In the twentieth century in the United States, a further shift in attitude toward government intervention occurred, in which government began to be regarded as the provider of public goods—services for overall well-being, but which, for various reasons, were not being provided within the private marketplace. Despite this more recent recognition of the legitimacy of the role of government as a provider of pubic goods through social policy formulation and execution, the ideological bias in the United States toward capitalism and private markets as the preferred service-delivery mechanism remains strong.

The view of government as a counterweight to other powerful forces in the society and the provider of last resort for certain types of services, although it had been considered at an earlier point in many European societies, is still not completely accepted within the United States. Given this orientation, health care services have traditionally been provided through a partially competitive marketplace in the United States; and, until recently, most physicians worked in small independent practices in which they could be viewed as a specialized type of small business (Starr, 1982). Only since 1964 has the federal government played a more major role in the provision of health care services to certain specialized groups, such as some of the poor and the elderly. In the last ten years, the United States has engaged in a policy debate over how to extend at least minimal health care services to all and whether the provision of these services should best continue as part of a private market, subsidized market, or a national health care system. The debate about the appropriate role of government in a capitalist economy continues to reverberate within health policy forums. As stated earlier and is to be discussed in more detail later in this book, no major legislation to reform the U.S. health care delivery system was passed as part of the health care reform debate during the first term of the Clinton presidency.

The Federal System

In addition to the basic philosophical underpinnings of the U.S. system, compared to many other countries in the world we have a more complicated system of government for policy formulation and passage. This stems from the federal system of government, created by the U.S. Constitution. Initially, federalism was a legal concept that defined the constitutional division of authority between the federal government and the state. Federalism stressed the independence of each level of government from the other, while incorporating the concept that some functions—

such as foreign policy—were the exclusive province of the central government, while others (including, importantly, health care) were the responsibility of regional units such as states. This model of government differs from both a unitary state (regional and local authority derive legally from the central government) and a confederation (national government has limited authority and does not reach individual citizens directly).

This notion of the partial autonomy of subnational units has long historical roots in the United States. While a major war (the Civil War) resolved the most vexing problem created by federalism (whether states can withdraw from the union), many issues remain today and continue to cause problems with health policy issues. No program better illustrates some of the difficulties of federalism in action than Medicaid, a joint federal-state program in which the units of government share fiscal and administrative oversight. A disjunction often occurs between the two units of government, so that a cutback or an increase in mandated eligibility at the federal level will cause a state to have to adjust to these budgetary and administrative issues (Lee and Benjamin, 1993; Reagan, 1972). In the last 15 years, as eligibility for Medicaid was expanded at certain points, states found that they had to find the dollars in the state budget to meet the entitlement of Medicaid and the Medicaid "match," as these funds are often called. The Medicaid match dollars have become, along with prisons, the most rapidly rising portion of expenditures in many states.

Because the capacity of states to raise taxes is more limited than is that of the federal government, problems from this type of arrangement have multiplied over the years—leading, in a related policy area, to the recent welfare reforms that will provide somewhat greater autonomy to states in setting policies for welfare eligibility and benefits, within federal guidelines. The federal system of government, by its very structure, produces difficulties in policy implementation across the boundaries of its different levels.

In addition to the complexity that the federal system creates across levels of government, limitations exist in other ways as well. As has been pointed out by experts on the founding of the United States and its governmental system, American constitutionalism goes beyond the general idea of a government of laws. It also includes notions of limited government, embodied within the Constitution and representing the fears of the founders of the Republic that a powerful central government represented a threat to the rights of individuals (Diamond, 1981). One aspect of this constitutional limitation is the important role of the states, and one of the ways that is written into the Constitution is through the *reserve clause*, which provides that any powers not explicitly given to the federal government are reserved for the states.

Another important constitutional limitation on the overall power of government was the division of powers across the three different branches of government. As compared to a parliamentary system of government such as is found in Great Britain, in which the head of government (the executive, known as the Prime Minister) is by definition part of the legislative branch, as are other members of the administrative group, in the United States the three branches of government (executive, legislative, and judicial) are separate and equal in their powers. The head of the executive branch (the president) is separately elected, and thus one can have a president from one major political party and a legislature controlled by the other party (in the case of the 1996 election, this is true for both the Senate and House of Representatives, who together form the Congress of the United States). This creates another impediment to a strong government, in that any given elected executive is not as likely to be able to have a personal program of new policies adopted by the legislative branch. Currently, many political experts and analysts argue that Americans prefer having divided government (a president of one party and Congress controlled by the other party) as a check on the power of the government.

Moreover, the presence of two different legislative bodies, the House of Representatives (whose membership comes from districts created in each state that are in proportion to the percentage of the population of the United States) and the Senate (whose membership consists of two representatives from each state), further dilutes power and makes it more difficult for new policies to be enacted. This was not accidental, but, as with the creation of reserved powers for the states, was the result of a compromise between the large and small states at the time of the writing of the Constitution. As a result of the creation of two different legislative branches, one in which the rights of small states were protected, the small states agreed to the passage of the Constitution despite their fears of being overwhelmed in decisions by the larger states. The two branches, however, create a further opportunity for divided and weakened government, so that even if the party of the president wins a majority in one of the houses of the legislature, it still does not have a majority in both, thus making it more difficult for new ideas to become approved legislation. Both the division of power among units of government and the division of power among branches of government creates what some experts have described as an institutional structure that makes efforts by progressive reformers much harder to achieve than would be the case under a different structure.

POLICY FORMULATION, IMPLEMENTATION, AND MODIFICATION: AN OVERALL MODEL

A number of experts in health care policy and health services research have described the public policy-making process and health care in the United States as a continuous circular gaming system (Longest, 1994; Torrens and Williams, 1993). In an approach that looks at the whole U.S. health care system, rises in health care costs are seen as setting off concerns among insurance programs and employers that force them to attempt to contain health care expenditures. These then have an impact upon the providers of care, especially hospitals and physicians who find their sources of revenue being constrained; they then try to take other actions that directly affect consumers of care, as individual patients, communities, and employees in workforces. At some point, the dissatisfaction of these groups may have an impact upon the political system and lead to widespread discussions of both health care crises and the need for reform (Torrens and Williams, 1993). This circular system of dissatisfaction mostly passes along the effects of one particular set of changes to another part of the system, resulting in a continuum that encourages each individual participant to figure out how to play the "game." For the most part major solutions are not encouraged. Torrens and Williams focus on unique aspects of health care and its complexity that make it especially vulnerable to this lack of rational planning and policy development.

Longest (1994) posits a public policy-making model within health care that is also circular. He views policy making as an ongoing process in which almost all decisions are subject to subsequent modification. He views a number of factors as external to the system (such as biological, cultural, demographic, economic, and ecological inputs). Each of these influences 1) the policy formulation phase of agenda setting and development of legislation, 2) the policy implementation phase of rulemaking and policy operation, 3) the policy modification phase of feedback in the form of outcomes, and 4) perceptions and consequences resulting from the ongoing process that influence future policy formulation and implementation. This model also focuses upon the political nature of the process in its actual operation. Despite the hope among many people, including many health services researchers and public health experts, that policy making can be a predominantly rational decision-making process, this model includes an understanding that interest group preferences and influence, political bargaining and vote-trading, and ideological biases all play a role in health policy making.

Before discussing, in the last section of this chapter, some of the unique aspects of policy making in the United States and how they have placed limitations on the achievement of reforms, this section will review the policy-formulation, policy-implementation, and policy-modification processes. While the processes are clearly linked, as the circular models propose, we also can understand some specific aspects within each.

Agenda-Setting Policy Formulation

There are two major parts of policy formulation: agenda-setting and development of legislation (Longest, 1994). The way in which issues emerge from the mix of all possible concerns to become a specific problem discussed within the political system is the agenda-setting aspect. As with the discussion of the overall circularity of issues within the health care system, there are many possible ways for issues to emerge onto a political agenda. Sometimes particular events and attention to those events in the media create the agenda, as with the sudden emergence of AIDS in the public awareness. As news stories grew about the new disease and its concentration in certain locations, concern about a new killer emerged, AIDS received extensive public attention, and ultimately increased public funding was a result. Another example is the recent attention paid to the relatively small numbers of problems that emerged as a result of the release of women from the hospital within 24 hours of delivery of a baby. While the number of problems was not large, as a nation we are often very sensitive to issues relating to the health of babies, so that even a few problems captured the interest of the public. In addition, many women across all age groups have either had babies in the past or plan to in the future, and they had opinions that they should be able to exercise more options (such as staying overnight in the hospital) if they wanted to. Thus, the overall issue captured first the attention of the public, and then of politicians in an election year when both parties wanted to be able to claim that they cared about women and babies, resulting in legislation banning what became known as mandatory "drive-by" deliveries, in which the mother was sometimes not allowed to stay overnight at all.

The example of "drive-by" delivery legislation is a good illustration of a situation in which a rational model of decision making was not applied. In a rational model, the discussion would move from a definition of the problem, to development of relevant alternative solutions, to evaluation of alternatives, to selection of a solution. Rather than receiving detailed exploration of the magnitude of the problem and the various alternative solutions, politicians of both parties—led by the president acting as the chief executive—raised the issue to a place of high visibility on the political agenda; they then moved to a solution that would please the broad public, rather than necessarily pleasing those involved in the actual delivery and financing of services. The willingness of President Clinton to raise the visibility of this issue in an election year illustrates the influential role a chief executive can play in agenda-setting.

Another of the aspects most commented upon in the American policy area was not important in this issue: the role of interest groups, especially health care provider groups as an organized interest group (Chelf, 1981; Peterson, 1993). Often these groups, because they earn their livelihood in health and are very interested in health-related issues, are able to play an important role both in agenda-setting and in drafting of legislation. Clearly, HMOs (whose policies limiting the length of stay for normal deliveries were the target of consumer concern) would have preferred that legislation had not been passed and that they had maintained more freedom to determine what policies they felt were best and most economical. But in the rush of interest in the issue by politicians in an election year, the interest groups were not able to mobilize and have their influence impact on both agenda-setting and drafting of legislation.

An interesting example of the circularity of these processes occurred as another related issue generated public attention (and thus was raised to the political agenda) in the period right after the election. Some concern was expressed about a few HMOs who were requiring that surgery for the removal of breast cancer be performed on an outpatient basis. Some consumers were outraged, and hoped the attention to the issue would follow the approach of the "drive-by" delivery situation and would lead to legislation banning the practice. Instead, the HMOs responded quickly that they would explore the policy more closely and focus on quality of care and outcomes to allay the development of legislation. Both because of the fast action of the organized industry and the timing of the issue (right after the election, so Congress was not in session and the president was not looking for an issue that could be addressed quickly to illustrate to the voters his continuing concern about health, especially that of women), the issue did not move onto the political agenda, and legislation mandating a minimum length of stay for surgery for breast cancer now appears less likely.

Development of Legislation

As contrasted with agenda-setting—a process whose steps vary greatly depending upon timing and the issue itself—the development of legislation mostly follows a set pattern. The legislative process begins with proposals in the legislature (Congress at the federal level), generally called bills but sometimes resolutions. Many more bills are introduced into Congress each year than are ever passed. Those not passed die at the end of that session of Congress. Any senator or representative can introduce legislation. Normally, staff members play an important role in its drafting, as may organized interest groups in complex areas such as health. Bills can be introduced into only one chamber of Congress, or identical legislation may be introduced into both chambers (this is generally the process if the president is proposing legislation). After being introduced, bills are assigned to the appropriate committee in each chamber for further study and consideration. The majority party in each chamber controls the appointment of committees and chairpersons of committees, and the chairpersons exert great power within the legislative process because they determine the order and the pace of consideration of legislative proposals. Typically, hearings are held on proposed legislation, often by a subcommittee but sometimes by the whole committee. After hearings, the bill is marked up, that is any changes will be made to the bill in a line-by-line process. The bill is reported out to the full committee with jurisdiction over the topic. Following approval by the full committee, the bill is discharged with a bill report, which contains information about the history of the bill and the reasons the committee has decided to approve it. The next step is placement on the legislative calendar for floor action. At this point, a bill may be debated and amended (especially if it is a major piece of legislation and is controversial) or it may remain as it was reported from committee (this is the more typical process, and is a necessary circumstance in order for Congress to move along with its work in a timely fashion).

If a bill passes one chamber of Congress, it must be sent to the other one for passage. The bill will go through a similar process in the other chamber (referral to a committee, hearings, changes, and so on) and eventually reemerge to the floor of that chamber for a vote. Given the two processes, often the bill that is passed in each chamber is not identical. In that case, it must be referred to a conference committee, generally composed of ranking members of each chamber of Congress, to resolve the differences. If a conference committee cannot reach agreement on the wording of the bill, it will die. If they do modify the wording, the conference report is sent to each chamber; if members of both chambers accept the report (the modified bill), the bill is sent to the president for signing.

A president has several options at this point in the policy process. A bill can be signed, and thus become law immediately. A bill can be vetoed, and thus returned to Congress for further consideration. If a two-thirds majority in each chamber repasses the bill, it becomes law over the objection of the president (the overriding of a veto). The president may also simply not sign the bill. In that case, the bill becomes law in 10 days, unless it is near the close of the Congressional session. In that case, a pocket veto has occurred, and the bill dies.

If a bill is passed and signed by the president, the final product is called a law or statute. At the federal level, laws are first printed in a pamphlet form known as slip law. Later they are published in a list of all laws and eventually incorporated into the U.S. Code of Laws.

Policy Implementation and Modification

The policy formulation phase, especially the passage of laws, focuses on the legislative branch of government. In contrast, policy implementation brings greater involvement of the executive branch of government. The legislative branch retains an oversight responsibility, and the judicial branch may be involved if challenges to the new laws arise. Rule-making and policy operation are the two major parts of the policy-implementation process (Longest, 1994). Policy modification can be thought of as a separate step, or as a part of an ongoing process of operation and policy change.

Rule-making is one of the most important parts of the policy-making process because laws are generally brief and not detailed. Thus, rule-making becomes a major interpretation process. Rules are the mechanisms by which agencies provide detailed restrictions, regulations, and guidelines to congressional statutes in terms of broad, less-defined goals. The interpretation of the intent and nature of the statute by the administrative agency, through the administrative rules that the agency establishes, both gives the statutory law life and determines the extent and scope of impact (Warren, 1982).

Formal procedures exist for rule-making, as they do for passage of laws. First, the organization responsible for the implementation of the law must publish a Notice of Proposed Rule-making (NPR) in the *Federal Register*. The NPR is a draft of a rule or set of rules that are proposed. The publication of the NPR invites comments across the policy community and industries involved in the legislation. Often, changes will occur in the proposed rules. In general, the length of time between the passage of the laws and the rules should be fairly short. In a few well-known cases in health care, however, clarification of rules has been much slower. The Hill-Burton Act (also known as the Hospital Survey and Construction Act, PL 79-725), passed in 1946, included a provision that grantees provide a reasonable amount of services to the indigent. Not until significant court action occurred in the 1970s, almost 30 years after the passage of the law, were the provisions about free-care obligations clarified. After the Health Maintenance Organization Act (PL 93-222) was passed in 1973, the appropriate administrative agency (then the Department of Health, Education and Welfare [DHEW] and now the Department of Health and Human Services [DHHS] organized a series of task forces, including members drawn from certain interest groups, because they anticipated controversy over the rules (Longest, 1994). In the case of complicated legislation such as Medicare, the administratively developed regulations are vast in length as compared with the considerably shorter length of the enabling legislation. Generally, though, the clarification of rules is a fairly swift and simple process.

In recent years, the tendency of Congress has been to increase the number of laws devoid of elaborate detail and to word many laws in more general terms. The courts have recognized the tendency of Congress to delegate its constitutional authority to develop policy via the law-making process to administrative agencies, but they have declined to force Congress to be more specific in establishing details through statutory law, as opposed to administrative rules. Through a series of court cases that collectively have established the delegation doctrine and have become incorporated into common law, the authority of the Congress to delegate policy formulation to administrative agencies has been upheld. Beginning with the case *United States v. Curtis-Wright Export Co.*, 299 US 304 (1936), the courts have consistently supported the right of Congress to delegate rule-making authority to administrative agencies as long as Congress set some meaningful standards to guide administrators. In *United States v. Cable Co.*, 392 US 157 (1968), the courts expanded rule-making authority even further by vaguely interpreting "standards" required in Congressional law to direct administrators as anything mandating administration that is consistent with law as "public convenience, intent or necessity requires" (Warren, 1982).

The policy operation portion of implementation involves the actual running of programs and activities, as promulgated in the specific legislation. The most difficult aspect of policy operation occurs when the legislation is based on an inaccurate premise of how a program would actually work, or when more than one organization is involved in the implementation phase. The involvement of multiple agencies and often multiple levels of government often occurs in the health care field. With Medicaid, for example, the implementation of most changes requires coordination with each of the state agencies responsible for the administration of this joint federal/state program.

While rule-making necessarily precedes the policy operation stage, feedback can also occur between the two phases of implementation. As a new law is implemented, problems with the rules as specified may become clear, and modification of rules and regulations can occur.

In some ways, policy modification is a further development of learning from the experience of the initial implementation. But, as compared to the situation in which only minor modifications of rules are needed, sometimes, as a new law or policy is implemented, major flaws are discovered and new policies are developed. The gradual progression from one law to another has been viewed by political scientists as an important part of the public policy-making process in the United States. Lindblom (1959) has characterized this process as incrementalism, or the building on existing policies by modification in small incremental steps. Often important policy initiatives that are thought of by the public as major new programs, legislatively, are amendments to other pieces of legislation and thus part of the policy modification process.

In the Appendix, some major health legislation is summarized. Many of the critical laws listed are actually amendments to other pieces of legislation. For example, the Medicare and Medicaid programs, are new titles on the basic Social Security legislation. Medicare is Title XVIII and Medicaid Title XIX of these acts, and of course further amendments to these have been passed over the years. Many other pieces of health legislation are amendments to the basic Public Health Services Act, initially passed in 1944, which specified working relationships of the federal government with state and local health agencies to prevent the spread of communicable diseases. The Health Maintenance Organization Act of 1973 was an amendment to the Public Health Services Act, as was the National Health

Planning and Resources Development Act of 1974, which set up a system of state and local health-planning agencies that was later disbanded.

THE CHANGING ROLE OF INTEREST GROUPS AND THEORIES OF WHY POLICY CHANGES ARE DIFFICULT TO ENACT

Political scientists and health policy researchers have written about a number of different ways to conceptualize the overall policy-making context in health care in the United States. Several of the major approaches have already been mentioned briefly, including incrementalism and the role of interest groups. This concluding section will describe these in more detail, as well as several related competing approaches—culture, interests, and institutions (Steinmo and Watts, 1995)—that have been used to understand better why health care reform has always been so difficult to enact within the United States.

Interest Groups

The role of interest groups has been recognized for some time, and fits within models of pluralism as used by political theorists. Pluralism describes a set of values about the effective functioning of democratic governments. Pluralists argue that democratic societies are organized into many diverse interest groups, which pervade all socioeconomic strata, and that this set of interest groups prevents any one elite group from overreaching its legitimate boundaries (Lee and Benjamin, 1993). Interest groups have occupied an important place in the health policy arena. They have been viewed as one of the three legs of the iron triangle of policy formulation, the other two being the bureau or agency in the executive branch that administers the policy area, and the committees and subcommittees within Congress responsible for legislation and appropriations in that area. The relationship among the three actors has been a symbiotic one of mutual dependence. Interest groups need access to Congress in order to get legislation passed that is favorable to their group members, and to relevant administrative agencies to influence the rules and regulations created in the executive branch. Congressional committees need access to the administrative agency to perform the oversight function of policy implementation and to determine what policy development would be desirable. Members of Congress and administrative agencies use interest groups for information and to mobilize support for particular programs. While interest groups have no formal government position or power base, they have nevertheless been coopted into the policy process. As with bureaucrats, interest groups provide specialized knowledge and expertise in different areas of health policy.

Interest groups often take stands on health-related issues. They monitor the progress of health-related legislation through the congressional labyrinth of subcommittee hearings, committee hearings, floor debates, and amendments. Interest groups alert their memberships to upcoming crucial votes, often focusing on mobilizing group members to affect vote outcomes.

The role of interest groups in policy formulation can move beyond passive monitoring of proposed legislation to active initiation of new policies. Given the specialized expertise and knowledge of interest groups, they sometimes may propose innovative solutions to health-related problems. Interest groups can also play an educational role: They can inform their memberships and even the general public about the need for health policy changes. In this role, interest groups can facilitate general consensus-building for various health policy initiatives that they support.

Ginzberg (1977) has identified four power centers in the health care industry that influence the nature of health care and the role of government: physicians, large insurance organizations, hospitals, and a highly diversified group of participants in for-profit activities within the health care area. The clout of interest groups in health policy formulation, in contrast to some other policy areas, is enhanced by the relatively unorganized and inchoate citizen attitudes toward health. For the most part, citizens think about the health care system and health services delivery infrequently. Exceptions to this occur when a person is temporarily in need of health care or has a close family member or friend who has a chronic illness or needs health care. Another exception would include a person's being personally involved in the delivery of health care through employment in the system, but then he or she may form part of an established interest group.

The dominance of physician interest groups such as the AMA has been weakened over time. One example of this was a loss in the political arena—the failure of the AMA to prevent the passage of the Medicare legislation in 1965, which they strongly opposed and campaigned against in the media, through material in doctors' offices and through campaign contributions and other traditional forms of lobbying. Despite AMA's loss in the overall fight, Congress did ensure in the initial Medicare legislation that the law did not affect the physician-patient relationship, or how a physician billed a patient for a visit, so that physicians would be willing to participate in the system. Not until 1989 did Congress adopt a set of policies that began to reform payment for physician services in the Medicare program.

Interest groups within health care have been able to influence policy by forming political action committees (PACs) to raise funds for candidates or political parties preparing for elections. The number and impact of PACs have mushroomed since the 1970s because of the passage of campaign finance reform laws. Since the reforms established campaign contribution limits for individuals, amendments to the laws in the late 1970s allowed interest groups to distinguish between "hard" money (counting toward campaign contribution limits) and "soft" money (raised in other ways and exempt from individual contribution limits), and allowed soft money expenditures to be used for party building and opinion development. Some experts believe these reforms have actually increased the impact of interest groups on elections (Drew, 1982a and 1982b). In the last 20 years, health PACs, and especially the richest ones connected with the medical profession, have become major contributors in many contests, especially Congressional races. On the other hand, some experts believe the increased public interest in health may lessen the influence of interest groups. Also, campaign reform, if enacted, would lessen the influence of all types of interest groups, including those in health, and is again being discussed at the national level. One recent article argues that changes within the health care system are shifting the way health care policy works—from an iron triangle dominated by an antireform alliance of medicine, insurance, and business to a more loosely bound policy network in which a reform coalition might be able to have more impact (Peterson, 1993).

The interest-group argument is one of the competing explanations that Steinmo and Watts (1995) also consider in their discussion of why reform is especially difficult to achieve in health care within the American political context. They reject the argument because, although they accept the empirical evidence supporting the importance of interest groups within the United States, they reject the comparative evidence that all countries that passed national health insurance legislation did not have strong interest groups (especially physicians) opposing the changes. Moreover, they also point out, as have many other analysts, that some reforms have passed over the opposition of organized medicine, especially Medicare, and they cite a number of more recent policy changes of a more minor nature.

Incremental Reform

The incremental reform argument states that the political process in the United States is not one of broad, bold movements in most areas, including health care, but rather is characterized by policy changes occurring in small steps (increments). This approach argues that rarely in the United States does policy become modified in dramatic ways (Lindblom, 1959; Wildavsky, 1964). The incremental model has been developed further by decision theorists and also by Alford (1975), who described three different approaches to reform: market reformers, bureaucratic reformers, and a structural interest perspective. The first two approaches each lead to incremental reform. However market reformers want an end to government interference in health care delivery and greater market competition, and bureaucratic reformers want increased administrative regulation of health care to deal with inequities in market competition. Both are limited and incremental approaches. Alford thinks these two approaches are more readily accepted by Americans than the structural interest perspective, which does raise more fundamental questions about who benefits from current arrangements in health care in the United States.

Culture

Besides the interest groups argument and the incremental reform argument, other explanations for the difficulty of achieving policy changes in the United States include culture and institutions (Steinmo and Watts, 1995). The culture argument is used to explain why, in many different aspects of policy, including the lack of any guarantee of national health insurance for its citizens, the United States is different from most Western European countries and the other countries with a related heritage of being English colonies, such as Canada and Australia.Within the culture argument, there is a special focus on the unique political culture in the United States (Anderson, 1972; Jacobs, 1993; Rimlinger, 1971). These experts argue that America has developed a unique individualistic and antistatist set of political values, and these have biased the country against the development of a welfare state, including resistance to a greater role for the government in provision of national health insurance. Included in the explanation of the uniqueness of this country is a focus on the immigrant experience and the support this has provided for the continued commitment to the values of individual responsibility, personal freedom, and antistatist views. It is pointed out that many of the immigrants were fleeing oppressive political systems in Europe, initially, and more recently in Asia and other parts of the world. Arguments against this approach are that, in public opinion polls, Americans have consistently indicated support for some type of comprehensive national health insurance system for most of the post–World War II period, now almost 50 years (Steinmo and Watts, 1995). Also, individualism has not stopped the development of a massive and comprehensive publicly financed education system, a large interstate highway program, or a generous Social Security system. One difference in these cases is that reformers have managed to argue that the programs were supported by American values and were essential for national defense (in the case of the interstate highway program begun under Eisenhower in the 1950s).

Institutions

The institutions argument focuses on the notion that political institutions shape how interests organize themselves, how much access and power they have, and perhaps even the specific policy positions the groups adopt. Also, institutions affect preferences, and thus help to structure in fundamental ways what we can imagine achieving. This argument focuses upon some of the unique aspects of a federalist system of government that this chapter has discussed. It argues that the "game" of politics in America is institutionally rigged against those who would use government—for good or evil. James Madison's system of checks and balances, the very size and diversity of the nation, the Progressive reforms that undermined strong and pragmatic political parties, and the many generations of Congressional reform have all worked to fragment political power in the United States (Steinmo and Watts, 1995). Proponents of this explanation argue that it is the fragmentation of political power that makes reform in health care so difficult to accomplish within the United States. We will return to this argument in Part Three of this book, when we consider the health care reforms of the past 10 years, the failure of the Clinton reform plan, and what the future may hold for federally driven as well as market-driven changes in health care. The next two chapters in this section will review the overall federal government role in health policy, and the major legislation that provides the backdrop for the evolution of the U.S. health care system.

4 THE HISTORY OF FEDERAL INVOLVEMENT IN HEALTH AND MAJOR HEALTH-RELATED LEGISLATION

Federal involvement in health is a fairly new occurrence in U.S. history. While a few laws and special concerns were passed prior to the twentieth century, the bulk of the federal legislation that has health impact has been passed since 1900, and most of it has actually been passed in the past 50 or so years. This chapter first will review briefly the history of involvement of the federal government in health care and health concerns, and then review some of the major pieces of legislation that link to health. A more complete listing of major health legislation is listed in the Appendix. Arranged chronologically, this list incorporates the major health-related legislation mentioned in the chapter, such as the Public Health Act and the Social Security Act. It also includes smaller, earlier pieces of legislation such as those dealing with the Merchant Marine, food and drug regulation, training of personnel for health care professions, and the research infrastructure of the United States.

HISTORY OF FEDERAL INVOLVEMENT IN HEALTH

Neither public health nor health care was an important part of the role of the federal government in the period from the founding of the Republic to the time of the Civil War. Even during and after the Civil War, the role of the federal government in health was only gradually expanded although the Civil War did create a major change in the overall involvement of the central government in many activities, and gradually, these came to include health care. From the 1930s on, the role of the federal government expanded both generally and as related to health—first with the Depression, then with World War II, and then gradually with major programs to help support the building of hospitals, the training of health personnel, research into important diseases and health care concerns, and gradually to the provision of insurance and funds for health care.

The Pre–Civil War Era

Most books mark the beginning of federal involvement in health care with the passage of a law in 1798, the Act for the Relief of Sick and Disabled Seamen, that provided for health services for this group by imposing a 200-cent-per-month tax on seamen's wages to pay for their medical care (Kronenfeld and Whicker, 1984; Lee and Benjamin, 1993). Shortly thereafter, arrangements were made to care for sick and disabled seamen in most major coastal seaports, through the building of what became known as the Merchant Marine hospitals and, later, the Public Health Service Hospitals. The federal government also played a role in imposing quarantines on ships entering U.S. ports in order to prevent epidemics, and in 1800 legislation authorized federal officials to cooperate with state and local officials to enforce quarantine laws. In 1832, hospitals were also built at ports along major lakes and rivers.

The major health problems of this era were infectious diseases such as tuberculosis and pneumonia, as well as gastrointestinal infections; there were also outbreaks of cholera, plague, smallpox, and yellow fever. Because national health policy up to the time of the Civil War was limited to the imposition of quarantines to prevent epidemics and the provision of medical care to merchant seamen and to members of the armed forces, most active concern with health matters was at the local level.

Federal involvement in health through statutory legislation, as in any area of federal policy, must be supported by authorization in the U.S. Constitution. Federal powers in the Constitution were delegated, while remaining powers not specifically given to the federal government were reserved for the states. Specific clauses must be used to justify federal involvement in health.

The authority for the legislation just described and subsequent pieces of federal health legislation comes from three provisions in the U.S. Constitution. One authorization—the power to raise and support armies, to provide and maintain a navy, and to pass laws "necessary and proper" to carry out those powers—is the original authority for the Marine Hospitals. Today it justifies the funds for the military health system and the VA (Veterans Administration) health system. A second authorization is derived from the constitutional power of the federal government to regulate foreign and interstate commerce. The original mandate for federal officials to establish quarantines comes from this source. Also, much of the federal regulatory authority in areas such as control of food and drugs, occupational safety and health, and some areas of environmental health are justified by the interstate commerce clause. The third and most major specification covering federal involvement in national health policy is the general welfare clause, the most commonly used justification for federal involvement in health today. It is used as the authorization for medical research, major service delivery programs such as Medicare and Medicaid, and health staffing and training programs. How these types of programs are administered among several agencies will be discussed in more detail later in this chapter.

From the Civil War to the Great Depression

The Civil War was a major defining event in U.S. history in many different ways. Beyond preserving the union, the Civil War initiated an alteration in the nature of federalism in the United States. Gradually, the federal government became more active in many different programs, beginning, of course, with higher rates of taxation and expansion of the power of government to build a large army to fight the war. More importantly for health care, this era led to the beginning of federal aid to the states with the passage of the Morrill Act in 1862, which granted federal lands to each state and allowed the profits from the sale of these lands to be used for the support of public institutions of higher education. This was the beginning of the land grant colleges in the United States, and of many programs in nutrition, nursing, and later, medicine.

In this era, more of the impact of government on health was through state, rather than federal, actions, especially early on. Several health-related pieces of legislation were linked to the growth of immigration and fear about the resulting spread of contagious diseases. One of these gave the surgeon general of the Marine Hospital Service congressional authorization to impose quarantines within the United States in the late 1870s. Another act, passed in 1882, was the first general immigration law, which included federal medical excludability provisions and allowed federal inspectors to board arriving ships and check for diseases among immigrants, as well as for backgrounds of criminal activity or idiocy, and to verify the ability of immigrants to take care of themselves without becoming public charges.

At other governmental levels, most states began to establish state departments of public health, and by 1909, such agencies were established in all the states. Local health departments grew in size and responsibility in most areas. In 1902, a separate health act had been passed, clarifying federal health functions and recognizing the expansion of the activities of the Marine Hospital Services by renaming it the Public Health and Marine Service of the

United States. This act legitimized the dominant role of the federal government in public health by specifying a system of communications among state and territorial health officers. The surgeon general, the administrative head of the Public Health Service, was authorized to convene an annual meeting of state and territorial health officers in order to discuss major health policy initiatives and campaigns for the control of diseases such as trachoma (an eye disease), typhoid fever (a highly infectious disease transmitted by contaminated food or water), and pellagra (a nutrition deficiency disease caused by lack of niacin). Other state and local actions in this time frame included the expansion of state mental hospitals to most states, and the continued development of local charity hospitals for the poor.

A major piece of federal legislation passed in 1906 was the Federal Food and Drug Act. While the initial legislation was focused more on regulation of the adulteration and misbranding of food and drugs, with an aim of protecting the pocketbook of the consumer as much as the health, this act became the basis for most of the present-day regulation of testing, marketing, and promotion of both prescription and over-the-counter medications.

Another major piece of legislation was the Maternity and Infancy Act, also known as the Sheppard-Towner Act. Passed in 1921, this legislation provided grants to states to help them develop health services for mothers and their children, and it has served as a prototype of federal grants-in-aid programs in health. The Sheppard-Towner Act proved to be quite controversial, generating criticism and opposition from conservative groups and from medical groups such as the American Medical Association (AMA), who openly called it "an imported socialistic scheme." Adding to the controversy was a requirement that services provided under the act be available for all residents of a state, regardless of race. Massachusetts was so upset that it unsuccessfully initiated court action to have the act declared unconstitutional. This particular piece of legislation was allowed to lapse in 1929, although many of the functions were resumed under the passage of the Social Security Act in 1935 (Skopcol, 1992; Wallace et al., 1982).

Modest Expansion of the Federal Role: From the Depression Through the Eisenhower Presidency

The Great Depression led to major federal actions in a number of areas, including banking, federal employment, regulation of business, and the creation of the Social Security System. While the Social Security Act of 1935 was arguably the most significant piece of domestic legislation related to health passed up to that time, it did not include health care services for the elderly, although early drafts of the legislation had included such provisions. (They were removed due to the threatened opposition of the AMA.) The act did solidify the principle of federal aid to the states for public health and welfare assistance, as had been initiated by the Sheppard-Towner Act, and federal grants to the states were included for maternal and child health and crippled children's services (Title V), and for public health (Title VI).

The program for crippled children represented a new thrust in federal legislation. Included were demonstration monies that became the foundation of experience for amendments in later legislation covering innovative project grants. The program had both comprehensive and preventive aspects, paying for all related medical care for crippled children or children threatened with crippling conditions.

Title VI authorized annual federal grants to states for the investigation of disease and problems of sanitation, reinforcing the dominance of the federal government in its partnership with local and state governments on health-related concerns. By the end of the 1936 fiscal year, about 175 new local health departments were created as a result of the federal funding. In the next year, states were able to turn to the Public Health Service (PHS) for consulting services in areas of nutrition, dental hygiene, laboratory methods, and accounting.

Consumer protection in the drug arena was further expanded by the passage, in 1938, of the Food, Drug, and Cosmetic Act, requiring manufacturers to demonstrate the safety of drugs before marketing. Another program of the 1930s and early 1940s was a temporary one instituted during World War II to pay for maternity care for the wives of Army and Navy enlisted men. Some experts have concluded that this program was responsible for an improvement in infant and maternal health during World War II, and although it was discontinued after the war ended, its success nevertheless became a factor in later debates about both national health insurance and the passage of health care for those eligible for federal categorical welfare programs as part of the Medicaid program.

One major accomplishment in this era was the inception of a major role for the federal government in health research. Although the U.S. Public Health Service Hygienic Laboratory had been established in 1901 to conduct bacteriological research and public health studies, this small beginning was converted into the National Institute of Health (NIH) in 1930 with the passage of the Ransdell Act. This act, along with the ongoing activities of the lab, marked a departure from the originally limited federal role of providing services to merchant seamen or preventing epidemics. With the Ransdell Act, the federal government edged into general health activities and began a very small role in personnel training. The act provided money for additional buildings to house health research activities, created a system of health fellowships, and authorized the federal acceptance of donations for research on the cause, prevention, and cure of disease (Kronenfeld and Whicker, 1984; Strickland, 1978).

A second act also expanded the federal role in health research. The first categorical institute within the overall NIH framework was created as part of the focus on cancer, which was begun with the passage of the National

Cancer Institute (NCI) Act in 1937 (Raffel, 1980; Strickland, 1978). NCI was authorized to award grants to nongovernment scientists and institutions, to provide fellowships for the training of scientists and clinicians, and to fund direct federal government cancer research. In a break with tradition, the provision of federal funds to nongovernmental institutions and scientists became a pattern for a majority of federal support for biomedical research. After World War II ended, these expenditures grew greatly in size and will be discussed further in the next chapter.

A major separate federal involvement in the direct provision of health care services is that for veterans. Although some limited efforts to provide services to seriously disabled veterans had begun at the end of World War I, the Veterans Act of 1924 codified and extended this role of the federal government. That act extended medical care to veterans—not only for treatment of disabilities associated with military service, but also for other conditions requiring hospitalization. Preference was given to veterans who could not afford private care. In 1930, the Veterans Administration was created as an independent U.S. government agency to assist disabled soldiers, as well as to handle other veterans' matters such as pensions.

The Roosevelt administration was interested in the consolidation of federal health functions as part of an overall reorganization of the federal bureaucracy. In 1939, the PHS became a component of the Federal Security Agency (FSA); the FSA became the umbrella agency for many domestic social programs, including the Food and Drug Administration (FDA) in 1940. A major piece of legislation, the Public Health Service Act, was passed in 1944; it and some of its most important amendments, such as the Hill-Burton Act to provide for hospital construction funds, will be discussed in the next section of this chapter. Under the Eisenhower administration in 1953, reflecting the growth in the size and number of domestic social programs, the FSA was renamed and given department status as the Department of Health, Education, and Welfare (DHEW). During the Carter Administration in the late 1970s, a separate Department of Education was created, leaving federal health and welfare functions in the renamed Department of Health and Human Services (DHHS).

The Kennedy and Johnson Years and Expansion of the Federal Role in Direct Provision of Services

Many major federal health policy developments occurred in the 1960s. The largest, the passage of the Medicare and Medicaid programs as amendments to the Social Security Act, will be discussed separately in the next section. Other less major but important pieces of legislation included the 1962 amendments to the Food, Drug, and Cosmetic Act. These were passed in part as a reaction to the European thalidomide disaster, in which a new drug turned out to cause serious birth defects, especially to babies' limbs.

Although the drug was not approved for use in the U.S. market, the amendments specified that a new drug needed to be effective, as well as safe, before it could be marketed.

Other legislation of this time period included a number of disease-oriented categorical programs that provided specific aid, as well as some programs aimed at specific regions of the country—such as the Appalachian Regional Commission—or programs focused on specific catchment areas for health problems. Two important programs dealt with education for health professionals and mental health concerns. The Health Professions Educational Assistance Act of 1963 authorized direct federal assistance, mostly in the form of construction aid, to medical, dental, pharmacy, and other health professional schools, as well as scholarship and loan aid to the students in the schools. The grants were contingent on the schools' increasing their first-year enrollments, and thus were part of a policy of concern about lack of adequate numbers of health professionals. In the mental health area, the 1963 Mental Retardation Facilities and Community Mental Health Centers Construction Act provided assistance in combating mental retardation through grants for construction of research centers and grants for facilities for the mentally retarded. In addition, assistance was provided for construction of community health centers, which proved to be a major undertaking at a time when many states were beginning the process of deinstitutionalization from inpatient mental health facilities. The next year, in 1964, a separate Nurse Training Act was passed, which specifically authorized funding for construction grants to schools of nursing.

One interesting fact about many of the new programs enacted in this time period is that few of them, even including ones like Medicaid that are classified here as part of a direct provision of services, were directly administered by the federal government. Medicare was one of the very few exceptions. Many of the other programs involved grants to states or to private health-related agencies. Grant-in-aid programs (excluding Medicare and Social Security) grew from $7 billion at the beginning of the presidency of John F. Kennedy in 1961 to $24 billion in 1970 (Lee and Benjamin, 1993). These programs became the prototype of involvement of the federal government in health care. Federal funds for biomedical research, health personnel development funds, hospital construction funds, health care financing, and a large range of categorical programs all grew in this time period, attesting to an expanding role for the federal government in health care.

Controversy and Contraction in the Federal Role: The Unsettled Times from 1969 Forward

Attempting to divide the recent past into clear periods is always difficult. While there are ways in which to divide the years from 1969 to now (by presidencies would be one way, or by shifts in political parties would be another), this will occur more in the following chapters. This section deals mostly with the policies and laws of the Nixon administration, the brief Ford administration, and the Carter administration, or two Republican presidencies (one in which the president was not elected to the office) and one Democratic presidency. Chapter 5 will focus on some of the major federal programs enacted during the Reagan and Bush presidencies (or the period from 1981 through 1992), a period that saw a shift from the Democratic presidency of Carter. Part Three (or Chapters 6 and 7) deals more with the period from 1992 forward (the years of the Clinton presidency), and looks at future issues and changes in the federal role as the United States enters the twenty-first century.

One thing that has been true from 1969 to the present, given the failure of major health care reform in the first term of the Clinton presidency, is that it has been an era of controversy about the appropriate role of the federal government, as well as a period of contraction in some ways (often in response to the press of the growing federal debt and the need to constrain growth in all government programs, including health care). During the Nixon and Ford administrations, considerable conflict developed among the branches of government, especially between the executive and legislative, over domestic social policy. President Nixon coined the term "new federalism" to describe his efforts to move away from the categorical program focus of the Johnson years toward general revenue sharing. In revenue sharing, federal dollars are transferred into state and local governments (often through block grants) for many different purposes and with fewer restrictions (strings) than was the case in specific grant programs, which often specified that funds should be spent on a certain type of program (in the maternal and child health area, for example). Congress generally favored categorical grants with their detailed provisions and control, while Nixon pushed revenue sharing and block grants to states. The Nixon administration also, in contrast to Johnson, preferred actions in the private rather than the public sector. Categorical programs continued to grow, however, but in the health care area, the huge growth of the Medicare and Medicaid programs swamped all other policy efforts. Some major policy initiatives outside of Medicare and Medicaid occurred in the 1970s. Health personnel policy over the decade of the 1970s shifted to focus more on areas with special needs, rather than on growth in all categories and places.

Most changes during the Nixon presidency and the brief presidency of Ford involved Medicare and Medicaid, and attempts to control costs. (These will be discussed in more detail as part of the description of these specific pieces of legislation later in this chapter.) A number of the policies enacted in this period were designed to deal with rising costs, through placing constraints on payments, reviewing care to be sure it was actually needed, and early changes in the organization of care delivery. Early legislation encouraging the development of HMOs (health maintenance organizations) was the forerunner of today's growth in managed care.

There were some important programs enacted in the health personnel and health facilities areas, however. Federal subsidies of hospitals and other health care facility construction were ended, partially as a reaction to skyrocketing health care costs. In their place, some programs began to explore planning and regulatory mechanisms to control expansion of facilities. One such was the National Health Planning and Resources Development Act of 1974, discussed in more detail under amendments to the Public Health Service Act. Health personnel policies by the mid-1970s began to focus on specialty and geographic maldistribution of physicians rather than on physician shortages, and by the end of this period there was a concern about physician oversupply.

There were few new policy initiatives in health during the presidency of Jimmy Carter (1977–80), due both to some lack of overall interest in the issue and to the difficulty in having policies enacted (such as failed attempts to have Congress enact new hospital cost-containment legislation). By the end of the Carter presidency, the climate for expansion in government programs was further diminished. By 1980, antiregulatory pro-competition approaches were gaining in popularity at the national level, as were pushes to give more autonomy and control to state and local units, reactions to the centralization of planning and regulatory programs that had been occurring in earlier decades. The decline of planning, the interest in block grant mechanisms, and the desire to control federal expenditures in health care have been major themes of the Reagan administration and the health policy process in the United States from the beginning of 1981 to the present. The specific policies and legislation to deal with these issues are discussed in the next chapters.

MAJOR FEDERAL HEALTH LEGISLATION: THE PUBLIC HEALTH SERVICE ACT AND RELATED STATUTES

One major piece of federal health legislation, the Public Health Service Act of 1944, consolidated previously existing health legislation. Many early federal health statutes were later incorporated into the Public Health Service Act, including the Merchant Marine Seaman Act of 1798. The thrust of federal efforts in the merchant marine area started a trend of providing services to clearly defined and selected groups. This trend, which may be contrasted with universal coverage, has continued into the twentieth century with coverage for the elderly and the poor. Other aspects of the Marine Hospital Service were also consolidated, first in the 1902 Public Health and Marine Service Act and then in the 1944 legislation. Titles V and VI of the

Social Security Act were also incorporated into the 1944 Public Health Service Act, as were disease-specific legislation such as the Venereal Disease Control Act of 1938. Similarly, the early legislation establishing the National Institute of Health was incorporated within the PHS legislation.

Original Structure of the PHS

The scope of the 1944 Public Health Service Act was huge. The act revised and compiled previously existing legislation about the PHS into one statute. The legislation included five titles (subsections). Title I defined crucial terms. Title II specified the administrative structure of the PHS, which at the time was to be directed by the surgeon general—originally under the direction of the head of the FSA and, after 1953, under the secretary of the Department of Health, Education, and Welfare (and later the Secretary of Health and Human Services).

There were four bureaus in the original PHS: the Office of the Surgeon General, the National Institute of Health, the Bureau of Medical Services, and the Bureau of State Services. Title II also specified grades, ranks, and titles of the Commissioned Corps personnel. Under this law, commissioned officers included not only physicians and surgeons, but also dentists, sanitary engineers, pharmacists, nurses, and other related specialists in public health.

Title III set forth the general powers and duties of the PHS. One duty was research and investigation into selected diseases and health problems, including the use of narcotic drugs. A second duty was working with state and local health agencies, especially for the purpose of preventing and controlling communicable diseases. Mandated specific activities included an annual conference of state health officers, provisions for the collection and compilation of vital statistics (birth records, death records, and so forth), grants to the states to assist in venereal disease control and tuberculosis control, and grants for the establishment and maintenance of local and state health departments.

A third PHS duty specified in Title III was the continued maintenance of the marine hospitals and the provision of services to merchant seamen and other eligible groups. The PHS was also to provide medical services to penal and correctional institutions and to federal employees for work-related illness or injury, and to provide medical examinations to aliens. Two additional nonservice functions were specified: 1) the regulation of the manufacturing, labeling, and sale of biological products related to the prevention or cure of disease (an incorporation of the earlier Biologics Control Act), and 2) the authority to conduct inspections, quarantines, and other procedures needed to prevent the transmission and spread of communicable disease. Care for those with leprosy and narcotics addiction was also specified under this title.

Title IV of the PHS legislation relocated the NCI to within the PHS, as part of the newly created subdivision labeled the National Institutes of Health. The Heart Institute was added as another specific institute in 1946, and now there are institutes to deal with most major categories of diseases, as well as ones linked to specific segments of life (the National Institute of Aging and the National Institute of Child Health and Human Development) and for general medical issues also. Title V dealt with miscellaneous regulations (Strickland, 1978).

Shifts in Organization

The basic legislation has been amended many times, with new responsibilities added and old ones deleted. The organizational structure has also shifted. In 1967, for example, five bureaus were created: the National Institutes of Health, the Bureau of Disease Prevention and Environmental Control, the National Institute of Mental Health, the Bureau of Health Services, and the Bureau of Health Manpower. Because PHS structure has reflected areas of concern within public health at various times, the 1967 changes reflected the growing importance of environmental and mental health concerns, as well as more traditional health and public health issues. Constant shifting and changing of the organizational structure and location of the PHS have continued from 1967 to the present, reflecting the crisis-oriented development of health policy in the United States. A typical response to a problem, either new or newly articulated, is to create a new bureau, restructure a bureau, or move a bureau around. Restructuring is driven further by the turnover of presidential administrations and political appointees within the bureaucracy. New administrations enter with fresh ideas about how to reorganize the bureaucracy in a hopefully more rational manner.

As an example of shift and change, the 12 years between 1967 and 1979 saw eight major reorganizations of the PHS and related federal health activity. (Some have continued as a major shift.) In 1968, line responsibility for public health programs was taken away from the surgeon general, the head of PHS, and given to the DHEW assistant secretary for health and scientific affairs; later it was given to the assistant secretary for health in the DHHS. Agencies such as the Food and Drug Administration and the National Library of Medicine were eventually incorporated within the PHS. Tracing all of these detailed shifts can become tedious, and it does not add to the overall themes of the specific legislation or the trends of the changing federal role in health care policy, but some more details are available in other sources (Kronenfeld and Whicker, 1984; Longest, 1994; Raffel, 1980).

Although many of the reorganizations have been designed to enhance rationality and policy implementation, the structural reorganizations have accelerated in pace and number since the mid-1960s. Working within PHS agencies in Washington has at times been very chaotic. Personnel have been faced with almost constant uncertainty about the programs they will be implementing and the personnel with whom they work. While some of these shifts and changes may be inevitable within government (and certainly within private-sector organizations, the last decade has been one of downsizing, reengineering, and reorganization that has been very difficult for many employees in such organizations, as well), stability of structure probably aids productivity.

The division of PHS least affected by organizational relocation and structural turmoil has been the NIH. Most of the changes there have led to the addition of new functions and new institutes in additional research areas. While the creation of each new institute has involved the movement of some grants and research away from older institutes, reorganizational shifts have been minimized compared to some of the non-NIH divisions. Not totally coincidentally, research promulgated at and funded by NIH has been regarded as one of the more successful areas of national health policy.

The Hill-Burton Act and Related Legislation

The Hospital Survey and Construction Act of 1946 (generally known as the Hill-Burton Act) was the first major amendment to the Public Health Service Act. This major piece of legislation was one of the first of several post–World War II federally funded health programs. Several different interpretations exist about the importance of this legislation and why it was passed. In the post–World War II era, many of the European countries passed legislation to reform their health care systems, as a reward to the general population for the toil of over five years of warfare on the European continent, as a way to address concerns about social equity, and as a way to deal with the lack of attention given to civilian needs and construction for civilian use during the wartime years. The United States had some similar concerns after the end of World War II. Very little hospital construction had occurred during the Great Depression and World War II, setting the stage for needed federal legislation to fund the building of hospitals. Many soldiers had received health services through the federal government during the war, and hoped to continue to receive health services in the postwar era. Many laborers had received health insurance benefits in lieu of raises during the war, since providing health insurance was one way to reward workers during the price controls of the war. Within the United States, debate about a more comprehensive national health insurance system occurred, with President Truman and the more liberal wing of the Democratic party preferring that type of legislation. Republicans and the more moderate wing of the

Democratic party wished to have less comprehensive legislation passed, although everyone recognized the need to increase the involvement of the federal government in addressing unmet health care requirements. As a compromise, after more comprehensive legislation failed to pass, the Hill-Burton Act became the major postwar initiative of the federal government. Senator Lister Hill of Alabama was a crucial player in devising the strategy of having the government provide funds for hospital construction, with the assumption that the private marketplace would be able to meet the less expensive needs of provision of health insurance.

The Hill-Burton Act provided grants to assist states to inventory their existing hospitals and health centers, and to survey the need for the construction of additional health facilities. After state surveys were completed, grants for hospital construction were available. Funds for surveys and planning were allocated to the states based on total state population. Federal funding covered up to one-third of the total costs. Funds for construction were allocated through a formula based on population and per capita income, and again covered up to one-third of the costs.

States had to meet several conditions to be able to receive funds. The law required the formation of state advisory councils that included representatives of nongovernmental and state agencies concerned with hospitals, as well as representatives of consumers of hospital services (at the time, an innovative expansion of representation on an advisory council). States had to submit a plan conforming to the regulations disseminated by the surgeon general for the construction of facilities, based on their statewide survey of need. One regulation that had little immediate impact but did establish a precedent for limits on health facilities construction with federal funds was a ceiling on the bed-to-population ratio.

The immediate impact of the Hill-Burton Act was considerable, partially because it was one of the first programs to pump large amounts of federal money in a visible fashion into local communities. By 1949, three years after the adoption of the Hill-Burton legislation, all states and territories had obtained approved state plans. As a result of the incentives in the act, most states had adopted licensing laws applicable to all hospitals in the state by the same year. Generally, state health departments became the administrative agency for the law in most states.

Many amendments to the Hill-Burton legislation were passed in subsequent years, extending federal financing for both hospitals and medically related nonhospital institutions. The Hospital Survey and Construction Amendments of 1949 increased the amount of federal funding available and increased the federal share of the cost of hospital construction to two-thirds, thus making it possible for less wealthy communities to benefit from the legislation. The act also authorized funding for research and demonstration relating to the development, utilization, and coordination of hospital services. The Medical Facilities Survey and Construction Act of 1954 provided grants for surveys and construction of diagnostic and treatment centers such as hospital outpatient departments, rehabilitation centers, and nursing homes, in addition to specifically naming chronic disease hospitals as eligible recipients of funds.

The 1961 Community Health Services and Facilities Act was passed as a separate statute, but included amendments to the Hill-Burton program that increased the amount of funds available for nursing home construction and extended the research and demonstration grant program to other medical facilities. Amendments in 1964 specifically designated funds for modernization of hospitals and gave greater priority to urban areas. Increased planning monies were also part of this amendment. Loan guarantees for construction and modernization were part of 1970 amendments. By 1974, the Hill-Burton amendment to the Public Health Service Act, along with its own amendments, became a new Title XVI of the Public Health Service Act.

Several noteworthy aspects of this legislation are its roles both in expansion of health care facilities and in planning in health care. Over time, the United States became a country rich in hospital resources. In fact, in the last 15 years, the Hill-Burton Act has been recognized as one reason for the current oversupply of hospital beds, as communities have changed and as the nature of inpatient care has shifted. At the beginning, however, this act made health care much more available across the country—including rural communities and smaller towns. As health care technology has increased, and transportation between places improved (along with the growing availability of automobiles to most families), the need for small hospitals in every community no longer exists. Today, as fewer hospitals are needed, it is more important to have facilities large enough to offer more advanced services and new technology. However, this current situation should not make us ignore the true benefits provided by the Hill-Burton legislation in the late 1940s in improving access to health care. Its role in initiating involvement in planning for resources is the other noteworthy aspect, and the impact of the legislation has been carried forward into the next two pieces of legislation to be discussed: the Comprehensive Health Planning and Public Health Service Amendments of 1966 and the National Health Planning and Resource Development Act of 1974.

The Comprehensive Health Planning and Public Health Service Amendments of 1966

As with so much of health-related legislation over the past 40 years, this act was also passed as amendments to the Public Health Service Act. Another name for this legislation is the Partnership for Health. This Comprehensive Health Planning (CHP) Act represented an important departure from much previous federal support in the health area. Prior to these amendments, categorical grants of designated funds for specific purposes such as cancer, dental disease, tuberculosis, and venereal disease were the major federal funding mechanisms. The Comprehensive Health Planning Act authorized block grants for public health programs, and also included provisions for the development of state and local planning for health services. Block grants were broader in focus than categorical grants, less bound to specific categories, and they gave state and local health departments greater flexibility in how federal funds would be spent within their jurisdictions.

The CHP amendments were a complete revision of Section 314, Title III, of the original Public Health Service Act. There were five major provisions under Section 314 after passage of the CHP amendments. To qualify for funds, states were required to submit a plan for comprehensive state health planning. Thus this legislation continued in a much more detailed manner the beginning of state and local planning efforts that the Hill-Burton Act required before federal funds were granted for building health facilities. Each state had to designate a state "A" agency, a reference to this section of the CHP amendments, to be responsible for health planning functions. Each state also had to establish a state health planning council, including representatives of governmental organizations and consumers of services. This council was required to have a majority of consumer representatives, and advised the state "A" agency. Another section, "B," provided grants to public or nonprofit regional, metropolitan, or other local area planning agencies, known as "B" agencies. These were local in force, in contrast to the statewide "A" agencies.

Other portions of this legislation provided grants for public health services, health services development, and training and demonstration. Monies were available to pay any organization to study health planning. State matches of funds were required for the public health services funds, including those dealing with training of personnel. Some additional areas covered under this legislation were grants to public or nonprofit agencies for services to meet geographically localized specialized health needs, and seed money for the stimulation and initial support of new health services.

The CHP legislation was amended in 1967 and 1970 and CHP planning extended. Local governments were required to be represented in the areawide planning agencies. State and local plans had to consider home health services, and assist health institutions to consider capital expenditures and to try to develop new expenditures consistent with the overall facility needs of the state. This legislation was replaced in 1974 with Title XV of the Public Health Service Act, the National Health Planning and Resources Development Act of 1974.

National Health Planning and Resources Development Act of 1974

This act amended the Public Health Service Act by adding titles dealing with both national health planning and development and health resources development. The act replaced a number of specific categorical programs, such as regional medical programs and Hill-Burton. In contrast to the 1966 legislation, national health policy guidelines were now required by the secretary of Health and Human Services. The guidelines would be implemented by establishing health services areas and health systems agencies (HSAs).

HSAs could be a unit of local government, a public regional planning body, or a special nonprofit corporation. The agencies had to form governing bodies with majority consumer representation. HSAs were to collect and analyze data, establish a health systems plan, and develop an annual implementation plan. These agencies were given much stronger powers than their corresponding agencies had been given in World War II. They had the authority to review and approve or disapprove of the use of federal funds within their respective areas for health services or resource development. HSAs were funded though grants on a per capita basis.

The state health planning and development agency (SHPDA) coordinated all health planning for the state, prepared an annual plan, and periodically reviewed all institutional services with regard to appropriateness. In addition, it administered a statewide health planning effort. All of these functions were specified in Title I.

Title II of the National Health Planning and Resources Development Act of 1974 provided assistance in modernization of medical facilities and for construction of new outpatient facilities. Also included was assistance for the conversion of facilities to provide new health services, to allow institutions to eliminate safety hazards, and to avoid noncompliance with licensing or accreditation standards. Also, the state SHPDA had to develop a state medical facilities plan separate from, but consistent with, the overall state health plan.

At the federal level, to increase powers for the planning agencies, Section 1122 of the Social Security Act, as amended, provided that hospitals and other Medicare providers had to meet all planning mandates. Failure to comply resulted in a disallowance of Medicare reimbursement for the portion of new construction or facilities expansion that was denied planning approval. This meant that local and state health planning agencies had authority to conduct voluntary assessments of health planning needs, to inventory existing health care resources and determine deficiencies, and, on a mandatory basis, to recommend and implement certificate of need (CON) and Section 1122 regulations.

Although this act represented a major increase in health planning, it still remained a limited approach with numerous deficiencies (Williams and Torrens, 1993a). The entire health care system of the country was "grandfathered" in. Planning agencies did not have the authority to effect facility or service closure. Secondly, extensive political involvement was inherent in the process. The ability of planning agencies to conduct and implement analytical and apolitical reviews was limited. Hospitals and other facilities with more fiscal resources were able to develop the most sophisticated analytical and planning documents and applications and, in so doing, to exercise greater influence on the political process. The attempts to increase consumer involvement, while laudable, were difficult to implement.

Some experts in planning and health policy have concluded that this planning legislation, despite its good intentions, actually resulted in complex and relatively ineffective planning processes (Salkever and Bice, 1979; Williams and Torrens, 1993a). Because of the lack of control over all health care resources and because of the need to focus on the encourage-ment of voluntary cooperation by providers, the overall planning effort was less successful than initially intended. Even the mandated aspects of the effort, the CON and the Section 1122 review, had minimal effect on the proliferation of health care resources, and rising costs continued as a major problem in the health care sector.

Thus this planning effort remained a subject of some controversy and con-tinued to be changed in small ways by minor amendments, but without dra-matically different results. The Carter administration actually began some of the push to weaken the already limited system, and major changes to this leg-islation occurred as part of the Omnibus Budget Reconciliation Act in 1981, under Reagan. HSAs received a reduced level of funding and were all allowed to accept contributions from health insurance companies. If a governor wished, he or she could request elimination of federal designation and funding in that state. The time limit for state compliance with certificate of need was also extended. Many previously required functions, such as conducting appropria-tions reviews, reviews of proposed use of federal funds, and the collection of data on hospital costs could be waived under the 1981 amendments.

As the 1981 amendments greatly weakened the role of the HSAs, they undermined their original function of areawide health planning. By the mid-1980s, a number of states had eliminated local HSAs and had devolved those functions to state-level agencies. (This lack of attention to and funding for planning will be discussed more in the next chapter, under initiatives of the Reagan administration.) The major focus of the Comprehensive Health Planning Act was to interject national planning and some coherence into a relatively haphazard and often barely existent system. The National Health Planning and Resources Development Act revised and strengthened this role, with an overall intent of moving the United States toward a comprehensive national health policy supported by an organizational planning structure, building from local to state levels of government. Over time, the HSA system became a major vehicle to control rising health costs and expenditures for new facilities, but one with a large role for the federal government. As politi-cal philosophies in the United States shifted to emphasize greater power for states and less centralization of functions at the national level, as well as less control by government at any level and greater reliance on the private mar-ketplace, the interest in coordinated planning efforts decreased.

Health Personnel Legislation

The federal role in funding training and development of health professionals grew from a miniscule one to a substantially greater effort by the late 1970s. However, expansion of the federal role ended and substantial retrenchment began with the Reagan administration. Its attitude toward social spending was congruent with a reduced federal role in health staffing and also was congruent with many health policy analysts' perception that earlier health professional shortages had been overcome successfully. By the early 1980s, many policy analysts even predicted an overabundance of physicians in the future.

Excepting temporary programs during World War II, the Health Amendments Act of 1956 was the first federal legislation that specifically addressed the issue of health personnel supply outside of the federal system. This 1956 act authorized traineeships for public health personnel and for advanced training of nurses. Formula grants to schools of public health were authorized in 1958. The Health Professions Education Assistance Act of 1963 provided construction grants for training facilities. Federal funding for training was expanded to include physicians, dentists, pharmacists, and podiatrists. Student loan funds were made available to schools of medicine, osteopathy, and dentistry, and were later expanded through numerous amendments to include other health areas, such as optometry, veterinary medicine, and medical technology. Special acts dealing with nursing and allied health were passed in 1964 and 1966. Modifications to these programs were included in amendments in the late 1960s.

Since the 1950s, federal involvement in heath personnel issues has consisted of grants to students and grants to institutions. One deviation from this pattern was the Emergency Health Personnel Act of 1970. That act authorized assignment of Commissioned Corps and other health personnel to areas in critical need of staffing, and provided the statutory basis for the National Health Service Corps (NHSC). The NHSC sent physicians and other health personnel to geographic areas experiencing doctor shortages in exchange for loan forgiveness, enabling students from less affluent backgrounds to acquire medical training.

The Comprehensive Health Manpower Training Act of 1971 expanded the federal role in training health professionals. Construction grants were extended, and special project grants and authorizations to health professional schools in financial distress were created. A new system of capitation grants was created for most health professional schools. To be eligible for these funds, schools had to increase first-year enrollments. Another extension of the federal role also aimed at increasing the supply of health personnel was start-up assistance to new schools of medicine, osteopathy, and dentistry. Loan provisions were broadened so that students who practiced for three years in areas experiencing shortages of health personnel could have up to 85 percent of their loans canceled. Scholarships for needy students were increased and special programs were created for geographic areas with physician shortages and for family medicine. Similar nursing programs were created by the Nurse Training Act of 1971.

The last major expansionary federal legislation in the health personnel area was the 1976 Health Professions Educational Assistance Act. Capitation grants and special project grants were extended to include schools of public health and graduate programs in health administration. Start-up grants, grants for schools in financial distress, and monies for special cooperative interdisciplinary programs were expanded. Medical schools continuing to receive capitation funds had to maintain previous levels of first-year enrollment, and, by 1980, had to have 50 percent of their residency programs in primary care areas (internal medicine, family medicine, or pediatrics). Restrictions were placed on the entry of foreign physicians into the United States. With this legislation, the federal role in physician training shifted from global expansion of the number of physicians to targeting of selected high-priority areas of physician specialization. As in other areas of national health policy, the Reagan administration retrenched the role of the federal government in personnel planning and training. (These changes are discussed in more detail in the next chapter.)

The Mental Retardation Facilities and Community Mental Health Centers Construction Act of 1963

Dealing with mental health has been viewed as a role of state government for many years in the United States. As early as the Colonial era, sections of jails were reserved for those with mental illness. Later, in the middle of the nineteenth century, Dorothea Dix and other reformers began the asylum movement to create special facilities for the mentally ill. By the time of the Civil War, most of the settled states on the East Coast and in the Midwest had state mental asylums. While these institutions have often come under attack as a result of the quality of treatment (as witnessed in popular movies such as the *The Snake Pit* and *One Flew Over the Cuckoo's Nest*), until the past 50 years, dealing with mental health issues was not viewed as a concern for the federal government.

Federal activity in the area of mental health has also been included as major amendments to the Public Health Service Act, although mental health problems were not included in the original 1944 statute. Congressional interest in mental health problems began with the Mental Health Act of 1946. That act included mental health problems in the grant programs of the PHS and established the National Institute of Mental Health. The Mental Health Study Act of 1955 provided grants for research into resources and methods for caring for the mentally ill. An amendment in 1956 authorized special project grants dealing with problems faced by state mental hospitals.

These previous legislative efforts served as important precursors to the Mental Retardation Facilities and Community Mental Health Centers Construction Act of 1963. Part of this amendment to the Public Health Service Act added mental retardation to the list of health problems addressed by the federal government. Substantial portions of the funds provided through this act were for construction for research or treatment facilities for the mentally retarded. While most states had some facilities to treat the mentally retarded, this statute initiated federal involvement.

A second part of this 1963 landmark legislation provided monies to construct community mental health centers. Few states had previously funded such centers, instead focusing their efforts on the large inpatient mental hospitals described as asylums in an earlier era of mental health treatment (or more pejoratively, by the public, as insane asylums). The 1963 act not only represented the initiation of federal effort in the previously ignored area of community mental health, but also created a whole new emphasis on deinstitutionalization of the mentally ill (Mechanic and Rochefort, 1990; Morrisey et al., 1985). Two years later, the act was amended to include grants (a 35 to 70 percent federal match, depending upon state income) to assist in meeting the initial cost of technical and professional personnel to staff the centers, recognizing that facilities without proper staffing were useless.

A number of amendments to the 1963 act that extended the types of problems and people covered were passed through 1980. In 1968, monies for facilities and personnel to treat alcoholism as well as for community mental health centers in rural or urban poverty areas were appropriated, as were monies to stimulate the development of mental health services for children. The scope of drug treatment services was expanded beyond narcotics to include drug abuse and dependence on any substance.

Mental retardation services were enlarged to include other neurologically handicapping conditions by the Developmental Services and Facilities Construction Amendments of 1970. Initially, federal community mental health centers were required to offer the five basic services: inpatient, outpatient, partial hospitalization (including day care), 24-hour emergency services, and consultation and educational services. Subsequently, the requirement was expanded from five to 12 service categories. A new emphasis on mental health services for the elderly was created. As in many service areas, the Reagan administration had new ideas about ways to deal with these problems in more general, rather than more specialized, ways, and these are discussed further in the next chapter.

Other Amendments to the Public Health Service Act

In addition to the major areas of health planning, construction, personnel, and mental health, the Public Health Service Act has been a catchall piece of legislation and a device for other federal health legislation in the post–World War II era. Often the changes illustrate the expansion of health programs on a categorical and noncomprehensive basis. The addition, subtraction, and merger of numerous specific programs have contributed to a frequent lack of overall coordination and coherence in health policy.

Amendments to the PHS have frequently created special programs for targeted groups or targeted health problems. In 1962, a special program of grants for family clinics and other services for migrant workers was created. In 1970, a categorical grant program was reestablished for control of communicable diseases including tuberculosis, venereal disease, rubella, and diphtheria. Also in 1970, the Family Planning Services and Population Research Amendments created an office of population affairs and authorized project training and research grants for all family planning services except abortion. The family planning programs became the major provider of health screening for low-income women and adolescents in the United States during the 1970s. In 1972, a special program of grants for screening, treatment, counseling, research, and educational services was passed for sickle-cell anemia and Cooley's anemia. The program was expanded in 1976 to include Tay-Sachs and other genetic diseases. An amendment in 1973 created emergency medical systems by establishing a program of grants and contracts to state and local areas.

Another example of a very specific amendment was the Health Maintenance Organization Act of 1973, which established a program of financial assistance for the development of HMOs (health maintenance organizations). The expansion of HMOs was advanced in this and subsequent amendments of the PHS through the provision of federal monies for feasibility studies, planning projects, and loan grants. The legislation established basic requirements that an HMO had to meet to be eligible for federal funds, such as provision of certain basic medical services, evidence of fiscal responsibility, and a policy board that included at least one-third enrolled members.

Another way the growth of HMOs was enhanced was through a requirement that every employer of 25 or more persons had to make available as an option an HMO in the geographic area, in addition to the traditional health insurance. Federal legislation nullified state statutes and regulations inhibiting the growth of HMOs—such as prohibition of solicitation of members over the telephone and requirements that all physicians in a geographic area be permitted to participate in the provision of any services offered by an HMO. While these provisions did lead to increases in membership in HMOs, those increases were modest during the 1970s.

The Social Security Act and Its Amendments

The Social Security Act of 1935 was part of the voluminous, landmark New Deal legislation passed in the throes of the Great Depression. The best known provision of this significant statute was to establish a retirement fund for eligible workers. Although generally the public understanding of the legislation was that it emulated private pension plans, the act, even originally, included significant welfare features. This act was the first major statute involving the U.S. government in social insurance, and represented a major increase in the role of the federal government as a granting source for the states. The Social Security Act included programs for the needy elderly, dependent children, and the blind. It also provided fiscal incentives to establish state unemployment funds, financial assistance for maternal and child welfare services, and additional grants to the states for state and local public health services. In 1950, the permanently disabled were added to the list of eligible recipients.

As with most large, complex pieces of legislation (such as the Public Health Service Act of 1944, discussed previously), the Social Security Act has been amended extensively over time. Many of the amendments greatly increased the role of the federal government in paying for the delivery of health care services. The first amendment that increased the federal role in paying directly for health services was the Kerr-Mills Act in 1960, which established a new program of medical assistance for the aged. Federal aid was given to the states to pay for medical care for medically indigent people 65 years of age and older. State participation was optional. The program became the forerunner of Medicaid and was implemented in 25 states before being superseded by Medicare and Medicaid.

The Social Security Amendments of 1965 established the Medicare program, the program of national health insurance for the elderly, through the new Title XVIII. The amendments also established a special program of grants to the states for medical assistance to the poor through Title XIX (Medicaid).

Part A of the Medicare program provided basic insurance protection against the cost of hospital and certain post-hospital services. Inpatient hospital service of up to 90 days during any episode of illness, and psychiatric and inpatient services for up to 190 days in a lifetime, were included. Extended care services, such as nursing home care, were covered for up to 100 days during any episode of illness. Some home health services and hospital outpatient diagnostic services were covered initially (and these areas were expanded over time with new amendments).

Part B provided supplemental medical insurance benefits and was a voluntary insurance program, financed by premium payments from enrollees, along with matching payments from general Social Security revenues. Initially, enrollment was very high (over 90 percent), and now it is generally above 98 percent, so that in practical terms, most elderly in the United States have both Parts A and B of the Medicare program available to them. Physician and related services, such as X-rays, laboratory tests, supplies, and equipment were covered, as were additional home health services. Both Part A and Part B physician and related services involved cost-sharing by the Social Security recipient in the form of deductibles and co-payments.

Claims and payment were not handled directly by the Social Security Administration, but were administered through fiscal intermediaries such as large health insurance groups, especially Blue Cross-Blue Shield, in many parts of the country. The Social Security recipient and the institutional providers, such as hospitals and nursing homes, were not reimbursed directly by the federal government, but received payments from the fiscal intermediaries in their geographic areas. Institutional providers had to meet conditions of participation, such as utilization reviews, that were aimed at ensuring a minimum quality of service. This program was an important departure from many earlier federal health programs in that it provided direct services to citizens, through a fiscal intermediary, but not through states and localities—as had been the case with many other federal health-related programs. It was consistent with the model of Social Security, however, in which direct payments were sent to individuals from the federal government, except that because health care services were very expensive and bills came in slowly after services, the initial decision was made to model payment after the major health insurance programs in the United States. At that time, patients did not receive the money directly and pay the health care provider, but rather health care providers sent bills to a third party (the insurance company or the fiscal intermediary), who then paid many of the bills. Medicare, administratively, was more complex in some ways than the earlier portion of Social Security.

The Medicaid program is even more complex in its administrative structure, although it follows a more standard pattern in health care of joint federal-state programs with a matching component in terms of funding. Medicaid was started as a program of medical assistance to public welfare recipients, with participation by any particular state being voluntary. Thus, from the beginning there was variability in coverage and amounts of services funded across the states, as well as in participation. By 1970, all but one state, Arizona, participated in the program. But not all states included all possible components—such as each category of medically needed services. States had the option of extending eligibility to the medically indigent—persons not on welfare who had a borderline poverty level of income but earned too much to be eligible for federally subsidized welfare.

Under Medicaid, all states were initially required to provide at least five basic services: inpatient hospital care, outpatient hospital services, other laboratory and X-ray services, skilled nursing home services, and physician services. A large number of optional services, such as optometry, were available for states to consider as portions of the program. States could also opt to provide more essential mental health coverage, ambulance transportation, and dental care, but were not required to do so by the federal government.

Amendments to the Medicare and Medicaid legislation began only a few years after the initial passage, with many having the goal of either extending the program or amount of services provided or modifying the institutional eligibility requirements and reimbursement schedules. The 1967 amendments featured expanded coverage for durable medical equipment for use in the home, podiatry services for nonroutine foot care, and outpatient physical therapy under Part B of Medicare, as well as adding a lifetime reserve of 60 days of coverage for inpatient hospital care over and above the 90-day original coverage for any spell of illness. Certain payment rules were also modified in favor of providers, such as authorizing payment of full reasonable charges for radiologists' and pathologists' services to Medicare patients.

More significant changes were incorporated into the 1972 amendments. Some new services such as chiropractic services and speech pathology were added. Family planning services were added to the list of basic Medicaid services. One set of changes increased eligibility in several important ways. Persons who had been eligible for cash benefits under the disability provisions of the Social Security Act for at least 24 months were made eligible for medical benefits under the Medicare program. Additionally, Medicare services were extended to people who required hemodialysis or renal transplants for chronic renal disease by declaring them disabled and eligible for Medicare coverage under Title XVIII. This aspect became known as the ESRD (end-stage renal disease) program. While this expansion represented a numerically small category of people eligible for Medicare coverage, the average medical expenses of these people and those in the disability category proved to be very high. At the time this provision was passed, some health policy experts believed this would be the model of expansion of Medicare as a form of universal health insurance coverage to more and more people—by adding various disease categories. However, the expense of the program and changing times and attitudes have resulted in no further expansions of Medicare based on specific disease categories. Moreover, the growing costs would increase concerns about both federal costs and overall costs in the health care areas in years following this 1972 legislation.

While it may appear contradictory, the 1972 amendments, along with the expansive provisions, also marked the first amendments to help control the growing costs of the Medicare program. Among the most important of the 1972 modifications was the establishment of Professional Standards Review Organizations (PSROs) to address problems of cost, case quality control, and medical necessity of services. Associations of physicians reviewed the professional activities of other physicians and practitioners within institutions. The use of PSROs by Medicaid was made optional in 1981, and later federal funding for PSROs was deleted. Another modification linked to cost control was the addition of a provision to limit payments for capital expenditures by hospitals that had been disapproved by state or local planning agencies, as a way to put some enforcement aspects into the health-planning mechanisms. Related to this was an authorization of grants and contracts to conduct experiments and demonstrations relating to increased efficiency in the provision of health services. Some specifically targeted areas for studies were: prospective reimbursement, benefits of ambulatory surgery centers, and payment for the services of physician's assistants, nurse practitioners, and clinical psychologists.

In 1976–77, a major reorganization of the U.S. Department of Health, Education and Welfare led to the establishment of a separate agency, HCFA (Health Care Financing Administration), whose job was to assume the primary responsibility for implementation of the Medicare and Medicaid programs. This new agency took over functions that had been located in the Bureau of Health Insurance of the Social Security Administration (Medicare) and in the Medical Services Administration of the Social and Rehabilitative Services (Medicaid), and made issues of administration of Medicare and Medicaid more easily centralized, but also more visible.

A major set of amendments dealing with fraud and abuse in both Medicare and Medicaid was passed in 1977. These strengthened the criminal and other penalties for fraud, included federal monies for state Medicaid fraud units, and required uniform reporting systems for participating health care institutions.

A specific set of cost-control measures was passed in 1978 to deal with the ESRD program, the Medicare End-Stage Renal Disease Amendments. Incentives were added to encourage the use of home dialysis and renal transplantation. A larger variety of reimbursement options for renal dialysis facilities was also included. Studies of the disease and its treatment were also funded, especially those focusing upon possible cost reductions in care for the disease.

The 1980 Omnibus Budget Reconciliation Act (OBRA '80) included extensive modifications in Medicare and Medicaid, with 57 separate sections. Many focused on controlling costs, although some also expanded services available—continuing the tradition of contradictions within the legislation—which generally leads to at least modest cost increases. Small rural hospitals were allowed to use beds on a swing basis for either acute or long-term care patients as needed. "Swing-bed" demonstration projects were allowed. The home health services provision of the Medicare legislation removed the 100-visit-per-year limit, but required that patients pay a deductible for home care visits under Part B of the program. The goal of these changes was the encouragement of home care over the more expensive institutional care. Some new services and providers were added, such as alcohol detoxification under Part A of Medicare and nurse midwifery under Medicaid.

The series of amendments to Medicare and Medicaid set the stage for the Reagan administration efforts in health, many of which focused on the Medicare and Medicaid programs. The changes in the 1970s had already demonstrated the differing concerns of cost containment, rationalization of care, expansion of some services, and the creation of new alternatives (such as the use of midwives under Medicaid) that might have goals of both an expansion and improvement of quality of care along with cost containment. They also demonstrated how these two programs became more and more the focus of health-related legislation from 1980 forward. For example, coverage for some mental health services, services for the disabled, and alcohol detoxification all were added to the programs through amendments, and they became ways in which two programs initially aimed at physical health care for the aged and for some groups of the poor addressed growing health and societal problems, such as alcohol abuse, drug abuse, and disability. Expansions, however, were never without costs, and cost increases, along with overall concerns about too large a role for the federal government in the lives of citizens and too high a growth of taxes, set the stage for a complicated period in health policy after Reagan was elected president in November 1980. More specifics of the Reagan era and how events of the 1980s led to the failed attempt at major health care reform by the first Clinton administration are the topics of Chapters 5 and 6, followed by a review in Chapter 7 of continuing problems and potential solutions linked to the role of the federal government in health care in the United States.

5 THE FEDERAL ROLE IN THE 1980s: THE REAGAN AND BUSH YEARS AND LIMITED, REACTIVE CHANGE

The Reagan administration both increased the pace of health-related policies and changed the overall orientation of the policies—from the emphasis of the Democratic era of Johnson in the 1960s but also of the Nixon presidency as well. Ford's short tenure in office was not one marked by large innovation in health policy areas, and ultimately, neither was that of Carter, although under Carter many pieces of legislation were passed to deal with minor changes in programs or to attempt to deal with rising health care costs. Some suggested legislation might have had larger impacts, but more innovative actions (such as a discussion, in the Democratic platform in 1976, of passage of national health insurance, under which Carter ran for President) never were pushed strenuously by the administration, most of whose concerns about domestic policy changes were subordinate to concerns over rising inflation in many areas and rising costs in the health care sector, specifically.

Some of the important aspects of the Reagan presidency as regards health care policy are linked to overall policy directions of the administration. A significant reduction in federal expenditures for domestic social policies was begun, including the elimination of revenue-sharing funds, started under Nixon, that had become an important source for local health care funds in some areas (Lee and Benjamin, 1993). Tax reduction was a major theme, and this resulted in significant increases in the national debt, and consequently a decline in the fiscal capacity of the federal government to fund many social domestic programs, including those dealing with health and health care. Connected to this reduction in social funding and declining federal revenues was decentralization of program authority and devolution of responsibility to the states, particularly through block grants, another overall theme of the Reagan years. One of the consequences that health policy experts have attributed to the use of block grants is an increase in inequities across states (Estes, 1980). Block grants give wide discretion to states in how funds are used, and this means that some states may fund programs for the poor and underprivileged, while others may fund broader-based programs. The end result of this is that it is harder to ensure uniform benefits for target populations, such as the poor and the aged, across jurisdictions, or to maintain accountability—because of a large number of varying state programs.

Other trends within the Reagan administration were more closely related to health care. These included efforts at deregulation and greater emphasis on market forces and competition to stimulate health care reform and eventually lead to more effective control of health care costs. However, the need to control health care costs rapidly became a pressing goal. The enactment of Medicare cost-containment efforts through the implementation of a prospective payment system for hospitals based on costs per case, using diagnosis related groups (DRGs) as the basis for payment, became one solution—even though it is a regulatory solution at odds with much of the philosophical orientation of the Reagan administration. This program is discussed further in a later portion of this chapter, as part of changes to Medicare and Medicaid enacted during this period. Other specific areas discussed in this chapter are health planning, health personnel, mental health, alcohol and drugs, and overall public health concerns, including concerns about health maintenance organizations (HMOs).

Despite the concern expressed about the need to increase access to health care in this country and the lack of equity across social and economic groups, some experts argue that the dramatic reduction in federal fiscal capacity due to tax cuts during the 1980s and the growing federal deficits in the same time period have had the most immediate effect on health services (Lee and Benjamin, 1993). The need to control overall government expenditures led to more attention being paid to containing rising health care costs in the late 1980s and early 1990s. The need to demonstrate how health care reform would neither cost more money nor hurt the effort to cut the federal budget deficit was one among a number of issues that became problematic in the debate over health care reform in the first term of the Clinton presidency. Despite a return to a Democratic president in 1992, the politics of limited resources had become a major political theme, one that focused on controlling deficits and thus the need to limit domestic spending of all types, including in the health area.

One thing that has changed in the format of legislation passed in the United States, beginning more clearly around the time of the Reagan administration, is the linkage between budget reform in the Congress and the legislative process. Major reforms in congressional budgeting were initially passed in 1974 as part of the Congressional Budget and Impoundment Control Act. Goals of this act were to coordinate congressional budget action and restore power to Congress vis-a-vis the executive branch. Before the reform, only the president, with the assistance of the Office of Management and Budget (OMB), formulated a national budget (Lynch, 1979). The Budget Act created budget committees within each house to hold hearings on the macroeconomic policy decisions and to set targets within 19 broadly defined functional areas, one of which is health. The act also set up a budgetary calendar. Hearings are held in the fall on fiscal policy needs, passage of the first budget resolution sets target spending levels by May 15, appropriation subcommittees meet in the summer, and by September 15, Congress reevaluates macroeconomic needs and makes needed changes in a concurrent budget resolution. A Congressional Budget Office (CBO) was created to provide an additional source of expertise and estimates. Several difficulties have occurred with the new budget process, and these began to have a major impact by the Reagan years and have, in some cases, become issues of great controversy in the 1990s.

What has been the impact of these budget changes? The results have been mixed, with some successes and some failures. The CBO has provided an additional source of expertise and estimates, and thus improved the quality of budgetary information available to congressional decision makers. Because it is a congressional agency, the CBO has not exhibited the bias toward presidential policies in estimates and information that has occurred in the past in OMB estimates. The new process has sensitized most members of Congress to budget considerations and constraints in a way that did not always occur before the budget reforms.

However, many conservatives initially supported the budget reforms as a means to control the rate of government growth and spending. In the initial years of implementation, the budget reforms did not lead to controls on government spending. One reason for this is what has become known as backdoor spending. Over the last 30 years, a large amount of total federal outlays (up to 75 percent of each year's budget in some years) has been removed from annual decision making because of the backdoor process. Backdoor spending includes contract authority by which officials can obligate the government to spend money in later years through legal contracts, borrowing authority such as legal obligations occurred in financing the national debt, earmarked revenues such as funds from a specific source (the gas tax that can be spent only on highways and transportation is one example), loan guarantees where the government promised to refund lenders in the event of default (such as some student and housing loans), and entitlement programs.

Of all these, entitlement programs have become one of the most complicated. While the next chapter will discuss some attempts by the Clinton administration to restrict certain entitlement programs, the growth in these programs in the 1980s was a critical element in increasing government expenditures. In an entitlement program, benefits are guaranteed at a legislated level to all eligible recipients (such as in Social Security and Medicare). The government is obligated to make entitlement payments to eligible recipients, even if insufficient funds were initially allocated in the budget. Because of Social Security Trust Fund programs (Medicare, Medicaid, Aid to Families of Dependent Children, and food stamps), over 50 percent of total federal expenditures were committed to entitlement programs by the middle of the 1980s.

In addition to the problem of entitlements, the reconciliation phase of the Budget Reform Act has created problems and changed the nature of legislation passed. The reconciliation phase was intended to modify the appropriations bill to make spending totals conform to the desired amounts specified in the second concurrent budget resolution. In the original act, only 10 days were allowed between the adoption of the second concurrent budget resolution and the final passage of a reconciliation bill. This quickly proved to be an inadequate time frame and prevented any real use of the reconciliation process. Because of this, in 1980, the reconciliation process was moved from the end of the deliberation on the budget to the beginning. This shift permitted the reconciliation bill to be utilized by authorizing committees to review and change legislation enacted in previous years. The impact of reconciliation at the beginning of the process has been to allow the adjustment of budgetary outcomes in response to political sentiment. Indirectly, this has restored some power in the budgetary process to the president and the executive branch by forcing trade-offs in funding for different functions. Without such a trade-off mechanism, interest groups could demand increased funding for their specialized areas without forcing reductions in funding for other areas. Because of this shift, more and more legislation from 1980 forward has been passed as part of a large piece of legislation—the Omnibus Budget Reconciliation Act (OBRA)—as can be seen in the Appendix in the years 1980, 1981, 1986, 1987, 1989, 1990, and 1993. In addition, related large pieces of legislation such as the Deficit Reduction Act of 1984 and the Consolidated Omnibus Budget Reconciliation Act (COBRA) of 1985 demonstrate this same trend. In the later part of the Reagan administration, the passage of the Emergency Deficit Reduction and Balanced Budget Act (better known as the Graham-Rudman-Hollins Act) established mandatory deficit reduction targets that further complicated the passage of legislation and had a significant impact on the Medicare program, especially in the last half of the 1980s. More recently, the passage of the line item veto, which allows the president to veto selected portions of overall legislation, may have a major impact on how new legislation is reformulated, but this act only began to become effective in the second term of the Clinton presidency.

HEALTH PLANNING EFFORTS

In the deregulation arena, federal health-planning legislation was not renewed in the 1980s, although other regulatory approaches were nevertheless used or even created (such as the DRG payment approach for Medicare). In accordance with Reagan's political philosophy that government regulations should be reduced, his administration greatly weakened but was not able to totally abolish the health systems agencies (HSA) system initially. In fiscal year 1981, the entire health-planning program was funded at $126.5 million. By fiscal year 1983, the funding level had been reduced to $58.3 million, a 54 percent decrease. For fiscal years 1982 and 1983, the presidential budget had requested the complete elimination of health-planning programs. However, Congress continued health planning at a low level of funding. With the exception of a few states where CON authority remains, hospitals and other health care providers are now able to enter markets at will, expand or contract physical facilities, and otherwise determine their own strategic plans, as part of a more pro-competition health care environment. In the Tax Equity and Fiscal Responsibility Act (TEFRA) of 1982, PSROs were modified, requirements for local HSAs were eliminated, and the funding was cut. The use of the new quality control agencies, the PROs (professional review organizations), was made optional in hospitals for patients under the Medicare and Medicaid programs.

From a philosophical perspective, the deregulatory attitude of the Reagan administration was grounded in a belief that the regulatory costs exceeded the regulatory benefits (Williams and Torrens, 1993a). Additionally, the Reagan administration was an advocate of the belief that the economic marketplace would be adequate for the achievement of social goals, without much intrusion on the planning side from any units of government, whether federal, state, or local. While there were criticisms of health-planning efforts up to 1980, by the end of the Reagan presidency, the lack of health planning was leading to expansion in for-profit facilities and greater closures of inpatient facilities. Pro-competition approaches have been followed at state levels as well, although more of them link to insurance reform in states than to Medicaid policies.

HEALTH PERSONNEL

As in other areas of national health policy, the Reagan administration reduced the role of the federal government in health personnel planning and training. The administration drastically cut funds for new scholarships provided through the National Health Service Corps (NHSC). Capitation grants to health professional schools were either totally eliminated or cut back severely. In the 1982 TEFRA legislation, capitation grants for schools of nursing and medicine were eliminated, while capitation funds for some other health professional areas were cut. The capitation grants for schools of public health and health administration were sharply curtailed. The student loan program was reduced from $13.4 million in fiscal year 1982 to $6.6 million in fiscal year 1985, a 51 percent cut. All nurse training funds were cut 26 percent from $65.9 million in fiscal year 1981 to $48.5 million in fiscal year 1983. Funding for new entrants into the NHSC was greatly reduced in TEFRA.

Many other changes were made in payment methodologies and approaches in the Medicare and Medicaid programs, and while many of these had direct effects upon health care personnel issues, further discussion occurs in the Medicare and Medicaid section, because the policy focus of most of those changes was to hold down health care costs, rather than to have a direct impact upon the numbers and types of specific health care personnel. The Omnibus Health Act of 1986 did include the Health Care Quality Improvement section, which provided immunity from private damage lawsuits for a professional review action that followed standards set out in the legislation. One major personnel-related piece of health legislation was the National Health Service Corps Amendments of 1987. This act reauthorized the NHSC and kept the idea of such a group alive within the federal government.

During the Reagan years, one important shift was to be concerned with the appropriate distribution of health personnel and a possible oversupply, as opposed to being concerned about the overall need to attract more people into health care professions and about a potential undersupply of health care personnel. Even for the highest level of personnel, physicians, by the 1980s, the consensus of health policy experts was that adequate numbers were being produced overall, although concern still existed about supply in certain specialties and willingness of physicians to locate in less desirable geographic areas, such as more isolated rural communities and some inner-city areas. The landmark 1980 report by the Graduate Medical Education National Advisory Committee (GMENAC) predicted an oversupply of most specialists by the year 1990. Predictions about the appropriate supply of physicians as well as new policy papers have continued to be discussed, and are part of the future issues that the federal government may need to deal with—such as the suggestions of the Pew Health Professions Commission of 1995 that would reexamine many aspects of training and estimates on numbers of various health personnel needed in the future (Pew Health Professions Commission, 1995; Schroeder, 1996).

One change that has been occurring in health care, especially in the last 40 years, is the growth in new categories of health care personnel, including physicians' assistants (PAs), nurse practitioners (NPs), and a whole array of technologists, aides, and other workers. Over two-thirds of all personnel now in health care are in allied health and support positions. Why is this change occurring? One factor many analysts would agree on as influencing the health labor force is changes in medical technology, along with special-ization and health insurance coverage (Aries and Kennedy, 1990; Banta et al., 1981; Starr, 1982). One unique aspect of the growth of technology in health care and its interaction with personnel needs is that new technology in health care often requires a new category of technical assistant to run the machine. This is unlike the trend in many production-oriented indus-tries in which capital investment decreases labor intensity. In the health care industry over the last 40 years, the greater the reliance on new equip-ment, the greater the need for additional support staff—although one trend now occurring in health care is to recombine the different categories of assistants within the hospital setting, sometimes as part of a restructur-ing of inpatient care analogous to the reengineering concepts occurring in other sectors of the economy. Some believe this type of restructuring may threaten the position and pay of registered nurses, one of the single largest health professions and a field that has remained between the 7th and 9th most numerous female occupations from 1930 to the present, despite all the changes in the economy, society, and position of women (Friss, 1994). These issues of health personnel policy, however, go beyond the scope of this chapter (Mick and Moscovice, 1993).

MENTAL HEALTH AND DRUGS

As with many areas of services under the Reagan administration, the Omnibus Budget Reconciliation Act of 1981 superseded all earlier com-munity mental health legislation and began a focus away from specific, detailed categorical programs to more generalized ones funded as part of block grants. The Reconciliation Act created two block grants to the states—one for mental health and a second for drug and alcohol abuse. As with all the categorical programs that were converted to block grants by the Reagan administration, the funds provided to states through the block grant mechanism were reduced by 21 percent from their previous levels under the categorical format. These cuts became part of a pattern of decreased federal emphasis (at least through specialized programs to deal with mental health services) on mental health concerns, even at a time when research and new drug therapies in the area were increasing in quan-tity, as was also the success of the therapy, to some extent. By the end of the Reagan administration, however, the growing emphasis on drug control led to an increase in the Alcohol, Drug Abuse, and Mental Health block grant, so that the amount increased $225 million from 1986 to 1987.

Mental health funding suffered in other ways under the Reagan administration. Although the Carter administration had helped to pass the Mental Health Systems Act of 1980 that established provisions for additional community mental health centers and authorized spending for new initiatives, the provisions were never implemented once the more conservative administration of Reagan (followed by Bush) was in place. The only aspect of this legislation to impact policy in the next decade was the creation of a President's Commission on Mental Health, which did produce a plan concerned with care for the chronically mentally ill that focused upon federal mainstream resources, especially those available under the Social Security Act (U.S. Department of Health and Human Services, 1980).

Mental health advocates remained active during the Reagan-Bush years, and some programs, such as the National Institute of Mental Health's Community Support Program (CSP)—a demonstration program for the care of people with severe mental illness—survived the decade, but not without repeated attempts by the Reagan administration to eliminate it. One successful new piece of legislation was the State Comprehensive Mental Health Services Plan of 1986, which built on the existing CSP system. The legislation authorized each state to work with the Medicaid agency and prepare a detailed plan for care of individuals with serious mental illness.

Advocates in the mental health area during the 12 years of the Reagan and Bush administrations focused upon improving funding in the already existing mainstream resources such as Supplemental Security Income (SSI), Social Security Disability Income, Medicaid, and Medicare. The national plan was for incremental change. Small structural changes were made in each of the four mentioned programs that increased benefits to individuals with mental illness in small ways, despite the lack of interest by the administrations in mental health issues—excepting those connected with control of drugs. During the 1980s, federal dollars accounted for 19 percent of the expenditures for both office-based mental health care and that in other settings, as contrasted to 29 percent for the rest of health care. As has long been true in the mental health area, the difference was met through greater involvement of state and local funds. State and local governments funded one-third of all mental health care costs, versus only 10 percent in the rest of health care (Manderscheid and Sonnenschein, 1990). Most of the federal monies came from the Medicare and Medicaid programs, and Medicaid payments were triple those of Medicare.

One bill that did receive support from the Bush administration and is impacting the future of those with mental illness and who are affected by substance abuse was the Americans with Disabilities Act (ADA), passed in 1990. Although predominantly a civil rights bill that protects the rights of individuals to employment and access to all public facilities, it also protects from discriminatory treatment in these sectors those who have been diagnosed with mental illnesses or with alcoholism. Given the stigma that has characterized these health problems, these protections are important in helping those in treatment to be more successful in remaining within the mainstream of American society, including retaining employment.

OTHER HEALTH AND PUBLIC HEALTH ISSUES EXCEPT THOSE LINKED TO MEDICARE AND MEDICAID

The Omnibus Budget and Reconciliation Act of 1981 (OBRA '81) included extensive budget reductions and program revisions for the Public Health Service. One major change was a movement away from specific categorical grants dealing with special programs and diseases to the consolidation of those programs under block grants. This was not an entirely new push, since some consolidation had occurred previously under the revenue-sharing approach. President Ford had once asked for budgetary consolidation of 16 various health programs, and had tied this to budget reductions, but Congress did not support the changes and Carter discontinued this consolidation attempt. When the Reagan administration came into power in January 1981, it decided to slash government social programs, including those in the public health area. The OBRA '81 legislation was the first step toward this goal. While the Reagan administration did not obtain its full request that 26 public health programs be combined into two block grants for public health, it did succeed in having 20 programs consolidated into four block grants. Six programs remained categorical.

Eight programs dealing with rodent control, water fluoridation, health education, home health services, hypertension control, emergency medical services, and rape crisis centers were consolidated under a preventive health services block grant. Similar consolidations occurred in mental health, alcohol and drug abuse programs (as previously described), and primary care programs. A maternal and child health (MCH) block grant consolidated seven categorical programs from Title V of the Social Security Act and the Public Health Service Act, including maternal health and crippled children's programs, sudden infant death syndrome SIDS, genetic disease services, hemophilia treatment, SSI payments to disabled children, and lead poisoning prevention and treatment programs. The six programs that remained categorical were: childhood immunizations, tuberculosis control, family planning, migrant health centers, venereal disease control, and an amount equal to 15 percent of the total Maternal and Child Health Services Grant that was to be set aside for use by HHS to fund projects of "regional or national significance" in training and research, genetic disease testing, and hemophilia diagnostic and treatment centers. The Women and Infant Care (WIC) program funded by the Department of Agriculture was also left categorical.

Maternal and child health programs have become a major area of expenditures in the overall public health arena. Expenditures for these programs were 47 percent of personal health expenditures in the late 1980s (Shonick, 1993). The percentages would be even higher if programs for handicapped children were included. One single item, the WIC nutrition program, a diet supplement program supported by the U.S.

Department of Agriculture, accounted for about 59 percent of the expenditures in this area.

One important aspect of the block grant procedure is that budget cuts were included with the block grant process. Total funding for the programs in each block grant was reduced by 21 percent. Given inflation, the real size of the cuts was probably closer to 30 percent. When combined with the simultaneous reduction occurring in state and local taxes in many parts of the country due to the recession, local and state health programs faced severe funding concerns. By 1983, Reagan's budget proposals included further reductions in federal grants in public health. In the 1984 State of the Union address, President Reagan proposed turning over 43 federal programs to the states and giving the states the option of continuing them or not. These changes were never enacted, however. Later on, funding for some areas was increased. The MCH block grant grew from $374 million in fiscal year 1982 to $478 million in fiscal year 1985. By fiscal years 1986 and 1987, the figure stayed the same as in 1985. In the Prevention block grant, inflation-adjusted appropriations decreased from $79 million to $64 million from 1982 to 1990. On the other hand, as AIDS became more important, funding for it also increased (Shonick, 1993).

OBRA '81 also included the elimination of federal funds for HMOs. All new HMO funds were cut out of the federal budget in 1982. This may seem a contradictory move, given the emphasis in the Reagan administration on a pro-competition model of health care, in which presumably HMOs would play a major role. In the early development of the HMO program, all parties—Democrats, Republicans, and health policy experts—had endorsed HMOs as an organizational device that would hold down rising health care costs and shift the focus of care to a greater emphasis upon prevention of illness. It was paradoxical that Reagan voiced support of the HMO concept while eliminating HMO funds. In fact, to the extent that the Reagan administration discussed ideal models of health care delivery, HMOs were a part of the orientation toward greater competition, since multiple HMOs in the same geographic area would be competing for customers. The stance of the administration, however, was that federal funds were unnecessary to stimulate this competition, and that private market forces would be sufficient to facilitate HMO growth.

Some other pieces of public health and other health-related legislation were passed in the early 1980s. The Orphan Drug Act of 1982 provided financial incentives for the development and marketing of orphan drugs—drugs for the treatment of diseases that affect so few people that revenues from their sales would not cover the development costs. In 1984, the Child Abuse Amendments involved infant review committees in decisions about the treatment of handicapped newborns, and established treatment and reporting guidelines for severely disabled newborns. In the same year, the

National Organ Transplant Act clarified a potential ethical concern in the health care system by making it illegal to acquire, receive, or transfer any human organ for money. In 1988, amendments extended this to a prohibition against the selling of organs or body parts of fetuses.

One growing concern in the health area by the mid-1980s was how to help people without health insurance. By this time, many health policy experts had demonstrated the strong link in the United States between employment and health insurance. One of the COBRA '85 rules was that employers had to continue health insurance for employees and their dependents who would otherwise lose their eligibility due to reduced hours of work or termination of employment for 18 months. This legislation helped people involved in changing from one job to another to keep health insurance during the transition period, although it did not address the concerns of people without health insurance through their current jobs or who were unable to find employment within a year or so.

Some reorganization shifts occurred within federal agencies at the end of the decade. In the OBRA '89 legislation, a new agency, the Agency for Health Care Policy and Research (AHCPR), was created to replace the National Center for Health Services Research and Technology Assessment. The new center continued the health services research priority, but expanded the emphasis on evaluation of technology and outcomes of care. A whole new program focused on assessing the outcomes of care was created to help explore issues of quality, effectiveness, and efficiency.

As part of a more general public health concern, as well as links to specific diseases, the Ryan White Comprehensive AIDS Resources Emergency Act of 1990 created special programs to distribute funds related to AIDS. Portions of this legislation drew upon old ideas within the federal government of greater inclusion of consumers in these decisions, perhaps due to the vocal activity and lobbying of AIDS activists. The legislation included a requirement that steps would be taken to involve the public in the process, and mechanisms for planning and evaluation were included.

One of the last major pieces of general health-related legislation before the election of President Clinton was the OBRA '90 legislation, which included the Patient Self-Determination Act. Health care institutions participating in Medicare or Medicaid (virtually all medical care institutions) had to provide all patients with written information on policies regarding self-determination and living wills. Additionally, facilities had to determine whether patients had advance medical directives. The goal of the legislation was to increase discussion and consideration concerning the conditions under which a person might no longer wish to receive certain medical services. While institutions are complying with the legislation by having patients sign additional paperwork, it is not clear that the requirement increases the real level of discussion about these issues.

The amendments to the Public Health Service Act again illustrate the turmoil and rapid changes that have occurred at times in both health legislation and health agency structure. Instability has undercut the development of a coherent and chronologically consistent federal policy. Often, shifts in administration (for example, the Reagan years) have changed the role of the federal government vis-a-vis states, local governments, and private health-related organizations. During the 1980s, the federal government moved, in a relatively short time span, from being supportive of HMOs through financial and organizational assistance to a more neutral role in terms of actual support (although the approach was still viewed positively by many in important health policy positions within the administration). While the federal categorical grant programs had encouraged local health departments to develop a multitude of specialized and separately organized programs, often independent of the state health department, the block grant procedure forced local health departments to work through their state units and encouraged consolidation rather than separation of program functions. These federally required rapid shifts in program focus and in state-local relationships have been deleterious to ongoing continuity in agencies and to smooth administrative functioning. Chaotic federal changes have led to a public perception that state and local health officials are ineffective managers whereas, in reality, the atmosphere of chaotic changes and crisis development of policy is federal in origin.

THE IMPACT OF MEDICARE AND MEDICAID REFORM

1981 and 1982 Reforms

As in many other facets of national health policy, the Reagan administration supported major legislative changes in Medicare and Medicaid. The majority of both proposed and enacted changes in Medicare were attempts to deal with the problem of health care costs. OBRA '81 was massive in its impact and the number of changes to Medicare and Medicaid, with 46 different sections relating to the programs. A number of provisions were deleted, including the coverage of alcoholic detoxification facilities and occupational therapy as a basis for entitlement to home health services. The Part B deductible on Medicare was also increased. In 1981, matching federal Medicaid payments to the states were reduced by 3 percent for fiscal year 1982, 4 percent for fiscal year 1983, and 4.5 percent for fiscal year 1984, although the cutback could be lowered by 1 percent in each fiscal year if a state operated a qualified hospital cost-review program, had an unemployment rate over 15 percent of the national average, and had an effective fraud and abuse-recovery program. Prior to 1981, Medicaid required states to offer recipients freedom of choice in the selection of providers. After 1981, states could apply for waivers of the freedom-of-choice requirements and could require Medicaid recipients to receive care from a specially designated pool of providers—the beginning of mandatory Medicaid HMOs for some recipients.

The TEFRA legislation of 1982 made a number of important changes in the Medicare and Medicaid programs. Co-payments for basic services, previously prohibited by federal statute, were made optional for states under the 1982 amendments for Medicaid. The regulations on acceptable error rates for Medicaid were tightened. For Medicare, hospice services were added as a covered service. In general, the most important changes were part of an effort to control rising costs. TEFRA set a limit on how much Medicare would reimburse hospitals on a per case basis and limited the annual rate of increase for Medicare's reasonable charges per discharge.

Creation of Prospective Payment

Even more major changes in the reimbursement policies of Medicare were passed in 1983. The Medicare prospective payment system (PPS), which based payments to hospitals on predetermined rates per discharge for diagnosis related groups—as contrasted to the earlier cost-based system of reimbursement that had been in place since the initial passage of the Medicare program—was created. In this act, Congress also directed the administration to study physician payment reform options.

The DRG payment system was a major break with how payment had occurred in the past, and was also a complex system that was regulatory in content. The federal government listed detailed regulations that explained how the new system would work, and forced hospitals that received Medicare funds (basically all hospitals in the United States) to completely rethink and redesign payment systems. For an administration committed to competition and the private marketplace as the determinant of the distribution of health care resources, this regulatory approach seems quite surprising. The Reagan administration, in this case, demonstrated that health care issues were less critical to it than many other policy areas. If rising costs in health care were going to make tax cuts and other policy goals of the Reagan administration impossible, then a regulatory strategy to hold down health care costs was acceptable.

The DRG prospective hospital payment reform system that was implemented by Medicare in the early 1980s did help to contain the growth in hospital costs to some extent. The rate of growth in annual hospital expenses slowed for a few years after the implementation of the DRG system, but then the rate of growth again began to increase. Some of the early fears about the implementation of this system were that hospitals would discharge sick patients too quickly, leading to unnecessary readmissions, and there was some evidence that this occurred during the early phases of the DRG payment system (Gay, Kronenfeld, Baker, and Amidon, 1989). Some reforms in payment for readmissions have occurred so that readmissions within too short a period of time no longer generate the start of a new DRG payment for that hospitalization. For the majority of patients, it no longer appears that access to needed care has lessened under DRG reimbursement (DesHarnais, Kobrinski, and Chesney, 1987).

There is evidence that, under the DRG payment system, hospitals have shifted more care into outpatient settings. (The revised payment approach applies only to inpatient care.) One way that hospitals can continue to maximize revenues is through more outpatient admissions. One survey of physicians found that, under PPS, hospitals have encouraged more outpatient testing (Guterman and Dobson, 1986). A recent summary of the impact of the DRG system argues that inpatient hospital care use declined initially and then stabilized from 1987 on, while outpatient hospital care continued to increase, as did costs for physician care (Edwards and Fisher, 1989). Thus the actual impact of the payment reform system on total costs has been less than hoped. As with so many reforms that affect only one payor and one type of services, there is much room for hospitals and other providers to learn how to "game" the system, that is, maximize revenue given the new rules. Many analysts contend that piecemeal reforms of the health care system generally lead to disappointing results after a few years.

Deficit Reduction Act and Related Changes

In 1984, the Deficit Reduction Act (DEFRA) continued to make changes in both payment of hospitals and payment of physicians. Further amendments for the rest of the decade also made changes in both areas, and other overall policy shifts.

The DEFRA legislation placed a specific limit on the rate of increase in the DRG payment rates in the following two years. The Graham-Rudman-Hollins Act of 1985 established mandatory deficit reduction targets for the five subsequent years. This had a significant impact on the Medicare program, leading to cuts in payments to both hospitals and physicians. COBRA '85 adjusted payments under Medicare for hospitals that served a disproportionate share of poor patients. Hospice care was made a permanent part of the program. PPS payment rates were frozen at 1985 levels for part of the year as a way to hold down health care costs, and payment to hospitals for indirect costs of medical education were modified. OBRA '86 continued the trend of reduced payments under Medicare, by altering the PPS payment rate for hospitals and reducing payment amounts for capital-related costs by 3.5 percent in fiscal year 1987, 7 percent in fiscal year 1988, and 10 percent in fiscal year 1989. There were also technical changes in the way in which outlier (extremely expensive) cases were reimbursed. OBRA '87 altered payment schedules for both Medicare and Medicaid. The wage index used to calculate hospital payments was updated, but the capital-related costs formula was reduced even more than had been planned the previous year, with reductions of 12 percent for fiscal year 1988 and 15 percent for fiscal year 1989. In the Medicaid program, expansion of services was included, with states required to cover eligible children up to age 6 with an option up to age 8. Additionally, the distinction between skilled nursing facilities and intermediate-care facilities was eliminated, and a number of features designed to enhance the quality of care in nursing homes were included.

Changes in 1988–89

In contrast, 1988 brought a large expansion in Medicare benefits, with the Medicare Catastrophic Coverage Act that included provisions to add coverage for outpatient prescription drugs, respite care, and a cap on out-of-pocket spending for co-payments by the elderly. The new benefits were to phase in over four years and be paid for by premiums charged to Medicare enrollees, including an income-related supplemental premium. This legislation was a major departure from previous policy making in the area of social insurance, because the expanded benefits were to be funded entirely by those who were current beneficiaries, and there would be overt redistribution among them. Despite being supported at the time by President Reagan, majorities in both houses of Congress, and the nation's largest senior-citizen interest group, the AARP (American Association of Retired Persons), the legislation was repealed less than 18 months later after enormous criticism (Himmelfarb, 1995). Wealthier elderly objected to paying the income tax surcharge and additional premiums; and many average-income elderly were upset to discover that what they considered the biggest need in the catastrophic coverage area—coverage for nursing homes and long-term care costs—was not included. Others failed to grasp what the extensions of the program would provide to them, even though the legislation would have benefited all of the elderly without supplemental coverage and might have provided those benefits at a lower cost to many of those paying for that coverage. As is often the case in politics and public opinion, perceptions matter—at times, more than facts. The pressure on Congress from both elderly constituents and interest groups increased, and the legislation was repealed before most provisions were implemented.

OBRA '89 continued minor, technical adjustments in the PPS and continued the 15 percent reduction in capital-related payments. The secretary of DHHS was required to update the wage index annually in a budget-neutral manner, starting in fiscal year 1993. A few new coverages were added, for some mental health needs and Pap smears. OBRA '90 continued the capital pay-ment reductions and reduced teaching adjustment payments permanently (they had been temporarily reduced in OBRA '87). A five-year deficit reduc-tion plan was included that proposed reducing Medicare outlays by more than $43 billion between fiscal years 1991 and 1995.

Physician Payment Changes

The other major area of reform within the Medicare program was to control physician costs, ultimately through a new physician payment approach. In 1984, the DEFRA temporarily froze increases in physician payment under Medicare, and mandated that the Office of Technology Assessment study alternative means of paying for physician services as a way to guide reform of Medicare. The act also created a differential between two classes of physicians under Medicare, participating and nonparticipating. OBRA '87 reduced physician fees for 12 "overvalued" procedures, and built in higher fee increases for primary care than for specialty care.

The major reform in physician payment was in the OBRA '89 legisla-tion. The Health Care Financing Administration (HCFA) was directed to begin implementing a resource-based relative value scale (RBRVS) for reimbursing physicians under the Medicare program with a four-year phase-in period. Thus this new system is recent, having begun in January 1992. The evaluative studies of the impact of the new system are not yet available. Moreover, most of this implementation is beyond the time frame of the Reagan-Bush administrations, the focus of this chapter. The RBRVS system has been a very controversial new policy. Physician groups launched protests in June 1992, when the initial draft regulations were first released. The AMA (American Medical Association) was so upset that it threatened to seek congressional action to change the proposed new system of reim-bursement (McIlrath, 1991a). Physicians argued that the reimbursement scheme was not fair and that transition rules were particularly inappropri-ate (McIlrath, 1991b).

The RBRVS system was initially developed by Hsiao (Hsiao, Yntema, Braun, and Becker, 1988). Previously, physicians had been paid on the basis of what their charges were for various services. In the studies preparatory to the development of the scale, how long it took physicians to perform various kinds of tasks was determined. Each service was assigned a relative weight based upon three geographically adjusted values for work, practice costs, and malpractice premiums. Thus new payment schemes were created related to the time and resources used. For the final application, a scale of relative weightings or relative values was formed as the basis of the new physician reimbursement system for Medicare patients (Hsiao et al., 1988).

Based on the complaints in reaction to the initial drafts, HCFA did revise the rules somewhat. Whereas the initial regulations would have increased slightly the fees paid to generalist physicians and decreased the specialist fees, negotiations with various groups from organized medicine, including the AMA, have been used as a basis for some modifications. By 1996, payments for family physicians were increased by almost 30 percent while payments for procedure-oriented specialties dropped by a similar amount (McIlrath, 1991a). Changes were gradual from 1992 to 1996. If prior payments for a service were no more than 15 percent above or below the determined RBRVS rate, the service was moved immediately to the new payment system. If the gap was larger, initial-year payments were a blend of RBRVS and the older historical payment system. In addition, the new system created an incentive for physicians to be full participating doctors who agreed to accept the Medicare rate as payment in full in all cases. Those physicians received a full payment amount according to the schedule, while physicians who did not agree received only 95 percent of the scheduled amount (McIlrath, 1991b). The revised rules issued in December 1991 actually increased average payment levels in 16 states and four specialties, as compared to no states and one specialty in the June 1991 draft. Thus the protests by physicians did lead to policy changes and some greater effort to seek cooperation with physicians (McIlrath, 1991b).

The evidence on how well the new RBRVS payment system is performing is not yet clear in terms of holding down cost increases, and the issue of its success in shifting the relative supply of generalist physicians versus specialists will take even longer to assess. This is because the pipeline between a person beginning to study medicine, choosing a residency and specialty, and then being in practice is at least 7 to 8 years, and often longer. Even then, the changes occur initially only in new graduates. Additionally, many in health care are concerned that a reimbursement change is also being used as a way to try to affect the relative distribution of physicians, without adequate public discussion. Specifically, many physicians feel there has not been an adequate public or professional discussion of the issues involved. The implementation of RBRVS has led some physicians to argue that the health care system is becoming increasingly bureaucratic, and is limiting the options for practice in the name of cost control.

Medical Policies and Overall Impact

One other reform included in the OBRA '90 legislation was aimed at simplification of Medigap policies, those policies that the elderly buy to supplement their Medicare coverage. Most of these policies cover some of the drug costs and the co-pays that are required by the current structure of Medicare. Before this legislation, Medicare beneficiaries had a choice of hundreds of Medigap policies, with widely varying benefits that were difficult to compare from one plan to the next. Because of the new legislation, by July 1992, all Medigap policies had to conform to one of 10 standardized packages developed by the National Association of Insurance Commissioners (NAIC). According to a study of the impact of this legislation, most consumers have picked plans that offer the best coverage of Medicare's basic cost-sharing requirements for hospital and physician services. Fewer consumers have picked the more expensive plans that offer additional benefits such as preventive care, at-home recovery, or prescription drug coverage (Medigap Reforms, 1996).

The Medicare and Medicaid reforms, especially the major ones on payment of hospitals and physicians, as well as other changes in the Reagan-Bush years, yielded mixed results as viewed from a policy perspective. Although the elimination of regulatory approaches was one goal, this was accomplished only in the health planning area. Especially in Medicare and Medicaid, the Reagan and Bush administrations used regulations to limit hospital reimbursement and physician fees. Even on a smaller scale, they used regulation to control the variety of Medigap policies offered so as to protect elderly consumers from purchasing worthless policies. Despite the talk about stimulation of pro-competition approaches, HMOs did not receive financial incentives and encouragement, and growth in this area was modest in many sections of the country during this 12-year period. The largest impact on health services came in this time period from the dramatic reduction in federal fiscal capacity due to tax cuts and the growing federal deficit, and initial attempts to control it. Congressional efforts focused on controlling cost increases through regulation rather than pro-competitive approaches. Even though the numbers of uninsured had been increasing in this 12-year period, access concerns were not a major policy focus, but rather most attention was given to controlling health care costs, partially because health care spending outpaced the growth of most of the economy through this period. As has often happened with a shift in political administration, the view of major problems in the health policy area also shifts gradually. The beginning of the Clinton administration was a time of growing concerns about access to care as well as costs, and attempts at large reforms, as discussed in the next chapter.

Part III
The Future of Health Care and the Role of Government

6 THE LACK OF SUCCESS OF MAJOR HEALTH CARE REFORMS IN THE EARLY 1990s: THE CLINTON YEARS

Concern over health care is not new in American society, although the amount of legislation related to health concerns has increased over fivefold in the last 50 years (since the end of World War II) as compared with the amount passed since the beginning of the Republic through World War II. Moreover, some of the major concerns of health care have existed for at least the last 25 years. Concerns about costs of care, quality of care, and access to care remain the big three issues of the U.S. health care delivery system. As the previous chapters have demonstrated, the decade of the 1980s (the era of the Reagan and Bush presidencies) was focused mostly on major concerns about costs of health care. While various experts and policy makers were at times concerned about access to care and quality of the care delivered, much of the legislation passed in that time period, especially the legislation related to the Medicare and Medicaid programs, focused on how to control rising health care costs. The picture of costs is well covered in many other sources (Angell, 1993; Rice, 1996; Schieber, Poullier, and Greenwald, 1992), including a more thorough discussion in earlier chapters of this book. The rise in health care costs has been slowing in the 1990s, although even in the recent years of slower increases, health care costs increased 7 percent in 1993 and 6.4 percent in 1994. Health care costs in the United States still far exceed those of other developed countries, especially when measured as a proportion of the country's gross domestic product. Yet, despite these large expenditures, universal coverage of the U.S. population for health care has not been achieved.

Most health policy experts as well as most politicians agree that it was the absence of guaranteed access to health care insurance and health care services that were part of the push for major health care reform in the beginning years of the Clinton administration. The push for reform is generally due to a coalescence of diverse factors. In 1992, these factors included declines in health insurance coverage, fears of unemployment and subsequent loss of health insurance, and a growing conviction by candidate Clinton and major Democratic party political analysts that health care was an issue which could help take back the White House for a Democrat—as well as growing interest in the topic by the candidate and his advisors as not only one that could win an election, but an issue that could define a presidency.

Besides the push for reform, this chapter will cover the most important aspects of the health care reform debate and the off-year elections after the failure of the health care reform plan. More specifically, the chapter will review the factors that led to the push for health care reform, the development of the proposed health insurance reform plan, the debate and failure of the passage of that plan, the 1994 off-year elections, and the health-related legislation that was passed after the 1994 elections.

PUSHES TOWARD REFORM

To understand better the political climate at the time of the first inauguration of President Clinton, the time when his push for major health care reform began to take shape seriously, this section will review each of the major pushes toward reform. These include: changes in health insurance coverage within the United States, fear of unemployment and the overall economic climate and its linkages to health care, the political pushes from within the Democratic party and those advising the presidential candidate that health care might be an important issue for winning an election, and the policy goals of the president that, at the beginning of the first term, focused on picking a major issue in American society and having a lasting impact upon it, both to help achieve the short-term political goal of a second term and to help achieve broader goals of having a presidency that made an important impact upon American society.

Changes In Health Insurance Coverage

Having good health insurance coverage is one of the most basic indicators of access to health care services in the United States. After the introduction of private insurance, issues of lack of health insurance coverage became a problem of special groups, such as the aged, the poor, and, more recently, the unemployed. Medicare helped to deal with access problems for the aged, and Medicaid helped for some of the poorest. Some later legislation (Consolidated Omnibus Budget Reconciliation Act of 1985) helped provide some transition in health insurance coverage for those people who were switching jobs, although at a substantial dollar cost to individuals.

Despite all these programs, some limitations on access to health care due to lack of health insurance was a problem even during the initiation and expansion of Great Society programs and Medicaid, but there is general agreement that the problem is larger today than it was in the 1970s (Andersen and Davidson, 1996; Friedman, 1991; Kronenfeld, 1993). Who were those in 1992 with limited access to care and who ended up in hospitals, unable to pay for their care (often called the uncompensated care group in discussions of hospital care at that time)? Typically, the uncompensated care population consisted of people with one—or some combination—of the following problems: poor health, poverty, and the absence of health insurance. Often, the presence of one of these alone brought minor problems in access, while a person with a combination of two or all three often had unpaid bills of thousands of dollars or may even have been a person whose health was ruined by delayed receipt of health care. The uncompensated care population included many young people; perhaps a third were children. Over half of those lacking health insurance were employed for at least part of the year (Cohodes, 1986).

While there is a range of estimates about the numbers of uninsured and underinsured people in the United States from the early 1980s on, most sources agree that there has been an increase in the numbers of uninsured since the late 1970s (Access to Health Care in the United States, 1987; Andersen and Davidson, 1996; Freeman et al., 1987; Kasper, 1987; Wilensky and Ladenheim, 1987). What are the trends in limited access as regards the uninsured and underinsured? The United States has always had many uninsured individuals. Traditionally, especially prior to the Medicaid program, income was a major determinant of access to care, especially access to outpatient and physician services. Several studies have demonstrated that the gap in levels of physician use between the poor and the rest of society has narrowed over the last 20 years (Aday, Andersen, and Fleming, 1980; Wilson and White, 1977). In many aspects of utilization today, the poor as a group actually use a higher number of services than do the nonpoor. On the average, the poor are less healthy than the nonpoor. This is true for many measures of acute illness and is particularly true for chronic illness. Thus it is appropriate for the poor, given their higher level of illness and resulting greater need for care, to utilize more health care services than the nonpoor. Disagreement has remained about the extent to which the poor may underutilize care relative to their need (Kasper, 1987; Kleinman, Gold, and Makuc, 1981).

In the late 1970s, the best estimates were that 25 to 26 million people in the United States—about 13 percent of the population under 65—were without health care insurance. The numbers of uninsured grew in the 1980s. Recent estimates ranged from a low of 22 million to a high of 37 million in the late 1980s. The source that estimates the figure as low as 22 million agrees that there has been a decrease in access between 1982 and 1986, the two dates of the studies, but simply arrived at lower figures in the earlier years and in the later years than did other sources (Access to Health Care in the United States, 1987). The Census Bureau had the highest estimate, 37 million, in the 1986 time frame (Moyer, 1989; U.S. Bureau of the Census, 1986; Wilensky, 1987; Wilensky and Ladenheim, 1987). In a recent review of statistics from 1980 to 1993, one source estimates that the uninsured population increased from 13 to 17 percent (Andersen and Davidson, 1996). Medicaid coverage increased (from 6 to 10 percent), but coverage by private health insurance decreased (from 79 to 71 percent). The proportion covered by private health insurance decreased for every age group, and the decline was especially noticeable for children under 15. Although Medicaid coverage for children has increased, as the review of legislation has shown, children still represent a higher proportion of the uninsured in 1995, compared to 1980. Another source has estimated that the numbers of uninsured increased from 27 million, 14 percent of the population in 1977, to 41.5 million, 18 percent of the nonelderly population in 1993. In the early 1990s, 14 states had uninsured rates higher than 20 percent of the nonelderly population (Brown and Wyn, 1996).

Who are the estimated 30 million or more Americans who have neither private health insurance nor coverage for health care services under public insurance programs such as Medicare and Medicaid? They are not a homogeneous group. While some are those whom we might assume are the major groups with the problem—the homeless, the socially dislocated—others are people who work in jobs either part or all of the year but have no health insurance coverage, or those who are temporarily unemployed. Surprising to some people, those without insurance even include some relatively wealthy families in which the primary breadwinner has a serious chronic illness, can no longer work, and yet is not a recipient of public health insurance programs.

Critical to understanding how some groups of people have no health insurance in American society is the realization that most private health insurance in the United States is purchased through employer-based group insurance policies. This represents about 85 percent of all private coverage. One major factor in the increase in the number of uninsured was the growth in unemployment in the early 1980s and again in the early 1990s. It is less clear why the rate of uninsured did not return to previously lower levels following the economic recovery and improvement in the unemployment rate in the mid-1980s. Possible explanations are shifts in type of employment (such as from manufacturing jobs to service jobs), shifts in the number of part-time versus full-time jobs, and Medicaid's failure to keep up with rising poverty levels. Some of the economic factors are discussed in more detail in the next section.

The poor and near poor are another major group without health insurance, with over 40 percent of the uninsured falling into these categories (some of these people are also among the working uninsured). Why aren't these people covered by Medicaid, the jointly funded federal-state program to provide health care services to the poor? Welfare coverage has not kept up with rising inflation over the last two decades and there are limitations on welfare programs based, in most states, on specific categories of eligible people. In 1976, Medicaid covered 65 percent of poor Americans, but this figure had shrunk to as low as 38 percent by 1983 (Mowell, 1989). As high rates of inflation hit in the latter half of the 1970s, most states did not raise their welfare eligibility levels to keep up with rising incomes and rising costs of basics such as housing, food, and utilities. In addition, many states provided limited or no Medicaid coverage for two-person working poor families, families in which the worker was more likely to be employed in the sectors least likely to offer health insurance.

There is another group of people with no insurance—those with a history of serious medical problems. Many of these people do maintain health insurance coverage as long as they keep their jobs. If they lose their current jobs due to the general economy or their health but can still work, they may experience problems in finding employment due to their health. Not only do businesses not want employees with illnesses that may require repeated absences, but increasingly, health insurance companies have underwritten "experience-rated" individual company policies. A workplace with a few high utilizers of health care due to chronic illness can raise the insurance rates for the entire company. Employers thus are reluctant to hire a worker who may increase overall costs in this area. While people who are medically uninsurable comprise a small portion of those without health insurance, they represent a much larger proportion of the uncompensated care expenses because they are very high utilizers of health services. Studies have estimated that 0.5 to 1 percent of the U.S. population is currently "medically uninsurable."

The Overall Economic Climate and Its Linkages to Health Care

Major shifts in the economy, many of which began to be noticed seriously in the latter half of the 1980s, led to growing concern about lack of health insurance and thus the need to reform the ways in which people acquire insurance for health care costs. Shifts in the major sectors of employment and shifts in the number of part-time versus full-time jobs are both related to ongoing changes in the economy. Many experts believe we are moving from a manufacturing-dominated to a service economy. A typical change would be illustrated by decreases in the numbers of people employed in automobile manufacturing (a group with extensive health insurance coverage), leading to increases in employment in fast-food establishments. Many of these jobs pay only the minimum wage and often are held by part-time workers who, typically, do not receive benefits such as health insurance. If the part-time worker is a high school student covered under parents' insurance or a person over 65 supplementing his or her Social Security income, the lack of health insurance provision in these jobs does not lead to an increase in the number of uninsured Americans. However, if these jobs are filled by heads of households or single adults who cannot obtain other jobs, there is an impact on the numbers of persons without health insurance.

Almost 17 million of the uninsured were employed more than 18 hours a week for all or part of 1987. Of these uninsured employed people, over half worked full time for all of 1987. About 43 percent, however, worked for firms with fewer than 25 employees. In one 1988 survey, 49 percent of uninsured workers were self-employed or were in firms of less than 25 workers (Health Insurance Association of America, 1990). Almost 80 percent of the uninsured were employed or dependents of employed persons in 1987 (Moyer, 1989). This includes workers in low-wage industries and workers in agriculture, forestry, construction, personal services, and retail trade. Agriculture is the industry with the lowest current coverage, with 16 percent uninsured throughout the year (Wilensky and Ladenheim, 1987). Individuals in low-paid jobs are less likely to be insured. In 1985, almost 70 percent of workers without coverage earned less than $10,000. Most of the rest earned less than $20,000. An analysis of the March 1994 Current Population Survey found similar figures, with 85 percent of the uninsured being working adults and their children, including 44 percent in families headed by a full-time employee and another 19 percent in families of full-time employees who work less than a full year (Brown and Wyn, 1996).

Data clearly point out some of the important linkages between the economy and health care insurance. As important as the real facts and data, however, especially for political processes, are how people feel about changes in the economy and linkages to health care insurance. The regularly employed middle class is now becoming anxious about health insurance (Starr, 1991). From the late 1940s through the early 1970s, stably employed wage and salary earners felt secure about increasingly generous employer-provided and tax-subsidized health benefits for themselves and their employees (Stevens, 1988). By the 1990s, as employers were trying to cope with both high health care costs and growing economic threats from foreign competition (especially in the manufacturing sectors), pushes for increased worker productivity grew. From this came discussions about the need to reorganize and even to downsize firms, with some employees losing jobs, and others being converted from regular employees with benefits to contract workers without health insurance benefits for themselves and their families (Skopcol, 1994). Union workers are finding that one of the most controversial issues in new contracts is retaining the existing health insurance benefits for themselves, their families, and retirees. These economic changes combined in the early 1990s to create political pushes toward an attempt at reform.

The Political Pushes

It is never clear at the time what events will push a new or revised political agenda forward. In 1990, while most of the trends described in the two previous sections about rising numbers of Americans without health insurance and growing fears of the middle class about not having health insurance due to changes in the economy were already recognized, nevertheless neither health policy experts nor politicians considered it politically feasible to talk about major governmental reform in health care (Skopcol, 1994). Certainly some major pressures were building. In 1991, the *Journal of the American Medical Association* published a special issue focused on the issue of caring for the uninsured and underinsured. But while these kinds of actions resonated within the health policy community, they did not lead to broad discussion among the public. Then, unexpectedly, in the summer of 1991, the type of occurrence described by policy experts as a "focusing event" occurred (Kingdon, 1984). Following the tragic death of Senator John Heinz in an aviation accident, the relatively unknown (but long-term political activist) Harris Wofford became the Democratic senatorial candidate in a special election in Pennsylvania against the better-known Republican Richard Thornburgh, who had recently been the attorney general under President George Bush. Wofford aired a television commercial during the campaign that argued "If every criminal in American has the right to a lawyer, then I think every working person should have the right to see a doctor when they're ill." This spot resonated with the public, and led to a focus in Wofford's campaign of calls for national health insurance. He managed to defeat his opponent, and the Democratic party began to realize that access to health care was an issue on the minds of the public.

During the Democratic primary debates, health insurance was a topic of major discussion. Several of the candidates developed well-thought-out, detailed proposals about health reform, especially Senator Robert Kerrey of Nebraska, who was in the forefront of interest in health care reform within the Democratic party. He introduced a comprehensive plan in July 1991, a year before the Democratic convention, when health care was just beginning to seem an issue of political appeal in the Wofford campaign in Pennsylvania. While Kerrey became associated with a maximalist position on health care, proposing a government-financed and government-run plan, other Democratic contenders adopted less comprehensive reform positions. The late Senator Paul Tsongas of Massachusetts, a friend of Harris Wofford since the two had served together in the Peace Corps, pushed an approach more similar to managed competition and the ideas of the economist Alain Enthoven—which later became publicly identified as the Jackson Hole Plan—based on the advice of Paul Ellwood, a physician who had years before been an early proponent of managed care. Managed competition envisioned a health care system that relied largely on market forces of supply and demand. Employers would pay a portion of their workers' coverages but would not necessarily be required to pay the whole insurance amount. The government would set minimal standards for benefits and help organize consumers into health insurance purchasing cooperatives.

Clinton was not particularly identified with the health issue in the early days of the primary campaign. After being pushed by his rivals, he released a ten-page health care policy paper before one of the New Hampshire primary debates in January 1992. The paper was not long on details, but was more in line with a "pay-or-play" type of plan that focused on health insurance provided at the worksite, with federal taxes to cover the unemployed or needy not covered by Medicaid. In later campaign speeches, Clinton also mentioned universal coverage, so that many experts interpreted his position as viewing "pay-or-play" as a transitional arrangement to a more comprehensive system.

By the summer of 1992, when it was clear that Clinton had won the Democratic nomination for the presidency, he and his aides realized that health care could be an important issue in the upcoming election. In his acceptance speech at the Democratic convention in Madison Square Garden in 1992, Clinton vowed "to take on the health care profiteers and make health care affordable for every family." This rhetoric provided a sense of direction and commitment to the public at large, but the campaign advisors were leery of providing more details. Campaign polls showed that voters wanted the system changed, but were not certain what changes would help them (Johnson and Broder, 1996). Other polls showed that Clinton was viewed by the public as the candidate who would do more to provide affordable coverage to all Americans. While some greater details were provided during the campaign (presenting a picture of mandatory insurance pools but dropping the pay-or-play terminology, which was under attack by Republicans), the overall goal of the campaign was to present few details and stick to rhetorical flourishes, much of which provided an "us versus them" theme of people versus the ingrained interests in health care. The ingrained interests were sometimes greedy hospitals, at other times greedy doctors, and often greedy insurance companies.

The Policy Goals of the President

Clinton won election in November 1992. How important would health care reform be in his administration? His political advisors differed on the best answer. A final election-day poll about the concerns of the voters ranked health care as only third in importance, far behind the economy and slightly behind the budget deficit. The same poll also presented voters with three alternatives for health care reform: a Bush-proposed subsidy plan, a single-payor plan more similar to the proposals of Nebraska Senator Kerrey, and Clinton's managed competition approach. Voters split among the three, with about a third in favor of each, although the least favored by voters was the managed competition approach.

Policy experts and politicians presented complex messages to the president-elect. Senator Jay Rockefeller of West Virginia cautioned against making too much of the Wofford victory in Pennsylvania. He argued that the lesson of the Medicare Catastrophic Coverage Act of 1988 was that voters will calculate carefully whether a promise of new health benefits is actually in their personal financial interest. Several pollsters argued that the American public believed the health care system was riddled with waste and greed, and that getting rid of bureaucratic waste would allow people to have all the health care they wanted without increasing costs too much (Johnson and Broder, 1996). Few experts in health care believed this, arguing instead that fraud and waste were not large, and that real choices might have to be made between regulation to control rising health care costs, competition as a different approach to try to hold down health care costs, and increased taxes for a government-sponsored National Health Program (Navarro, 1994; Starr, 1994; Thorpe, 1992).

While many aspects of health care reform created a potentially difficult situation for the newly elected president, some aspects of health care reform held enormous appeal. One of Clinton's aides, Atul Gawande, a 26-year-old Rhodes scholar on leave from Harvard Medical School so that he could work in a political campaign, advised Clinton that health care reform is "at once our most ambitious and our most treacherous task. . . . If health reform is passed and successful, it would be an indelible symbol of achievement and of your ability to create needed change in the face of special interests. . . . It would also be an accomplishment on the scale of Social Security" (Johnson and Broder, 1996, p. 94). This quote in a memo to the newly elected president clearly demonstrates the appeal that health care reform held for President Clinton. For a politician who thought of himself as a policy wonk, or detailed policy expert, who was concerned about how presidents are viewed by history and wanted to leave a lasting impact on the country, health care reform was the most challenging issue on the domestic agenda, and the one that would impact the greatest number of people. It was an issue about which everyone in the country shared some concern, as contrasted with welfare reform, which would impact a more limited number of people in the country.

INITIAL DEVELOPMENT OF THE PROPOSED HEALTH CARE REFORM PLAN

Given the importance of health care, it is less surprising that President Clinton decided to tackle the issue, especially given the enormous enthusiasm and optimism that followed the inauguration in January 1993. In this initial burst of enthusiasm, the president and his advisors, many of whom were relatively young and inexperienced in the politics of Washington and the national scene, forgot that he was, in some ways, a minority president, having received only 43 percent of the popular vote in a three-way contest with George Bush and Ross Perot.

What were the actions in the early days of the administration that helped to create the health care reform plan? Did any of these create major problems in the later attainment of this health care reform plan? Five days after the inauguration, President Clinton announced the formation of the President's Task Force on National Health Reform. The job of the task force was to prepare health care reform legislation to be submitted to Congress within 100 days of the beginning of Clinton's term. Hilary Rodham Clinton, wife of the president, was named head of the task force, and Ira Magaziner was named the operating head. Despite advice against the creation of the task force, against tackling overall health care reform as one big piece, and against appointing his wife as the head of the task force, President Clinton moved ahead with his plans.

Many of his former aides argue that in some ways Clinton's own intellectual capacities worked against successful health care reform. He was not inclined to follow the examples of more piecemeal reform efforts. He wanted a large impact, and he saw the interconnections among health problems. He wanted to tackle the entire issue. His mandate to the task force was to make the proposal comprehensive. Once a decision was made to have a comprehensive proposal, some group needed to draft the proposal and to do so quickly. On the surface, the creation of a task force seemed reasonable, if work was started quickly and a proposal was brought forth in a timely fashion (such as the first 100 days that has become a traditional "quick moving" time frame that takes advantage of the "presidential honeymoon" of newly elected presidents). One other advantage that Clinton saw for a task force was that it would remove any infighting among different cabinet secretaries who might claim jurisdiction over the area. The goal was to set up a system in which everyone had to participate, and in which decisions would come from the White House. As a former governor who had to deal in the past with HCFA (the Health Care Financing Administration) and its administration of the Medicaid program, President Clinton shared the opinion that HCFA and DHHS (the Department of Health and Human Services) were difficult agencies and were not popular with governors. The creation of the task force removed direct decisions from these agencies, and might help to create support for the proposal among governors. Clinton considered the support of governors (hopefully across political party boundaries) as important in building public support for the program.

Why Hilary Clinton was picked to head the task force is less clear. Some experts believe her role on the task force on health was modeled after her successful role in school reform in Arkansas, where she headed a task force that held hearings around the state and resulted in successful legislation to deal with educational problems. Others believe that it was a compromise decision, viewed as a more politically palatable way to provide some real responsibilities to the First Lady, but less dangerous than allowing her key roles in several different subject areas. In Arkansas, besides Hilary Clinton's leading role in the commission on education reform, she had led a rural health task force for several years and served as her husband's representative on a regional task force on infant mortality, in addition to serving on the Board of the Arkansas Children's Hospital and on the national board of the Children's Defense Fund. Thus health could legitimately be viewed as an area of partial expertise. Experts in the area such as Philip Lee (one of the architects of the Medicare program in the Johnson administration who returned to help lead health care reform under Clinton) became impressed with her grasp of the complex issues of health care (Johnson and Broder, 1996). Despite the qualifications of the First Lady in the area, it may not have been a politically wise decision, either for health care progress or ultimately for the reputation of the First Lady. Her placement in the position upped the stakes on health care reform, immediately signaling the importance the administration placed on the issue. Her presence may have diminished the willingness of some to critique issues and, thus, ultimately hurt the integrity of the plan. It also increased her visibility in a policy role, a visibility treated quite negatively by the press initially, and even more so as health care reform stalled.

Other aspects of the creation of the task force ended up being problematic. Certainly the decision to try for comprehensive reform made any plan more difficult to produce, but some experts believe that the creation of a commission ended up exacerbating this problem (Blendon et al., 1995a). The task force was cumbersome and large, making it difficult to meet and make decisions quickly. The notion that 500 experts, none of whom was identified publicly, would develop a proposal did not engender public support or enthusiasm. Because of the creation of the commission and the secrecy around its actions, the administration was not publicly perceived as gathering advice from either private-sector business leaders or physicians' groups, and thus the plan, when finally produced, did not carry the "aura" of endorsement from recognized business leaders or well-known physicians.

The political leaders in the administration were not naive about the immediate lessons of the past. They understood the importance of the "honeymoon" and the need to put forward a proposal quickly. However, moving the complex process of the task force forward quickly proved to be a daunting task. Despite the characterization of the beginning of the task force by meetings held at a feverish pace, going from daybreak until midnight, progress was not rapid. It was made even more difficult by the composition of the task force, which included as group leaders those recruited from the campaign. Participants in the working groups were often chosen for their technical knowledge, and many were regular federal employees on loan, members of congressional staffs, and academic experts on leave. Many were not true believers in comprehensive reform, and there was wide diversity of opinion, making agreement difficult. Yet the diversity was not wide enough to satisfy many critics, and private-interest groups such as the AMA and the press were unhappy at their exclusion from the panels. The press was also angry at the private meetings, even though most policy development in past administrations also had been held behind closed doors, and was even more secretive. The attempts at openness and discussion backfired in some ways, and the process proved slow, both due to an initial, deliberate separation of policy and politics and because leaks to the press resulted in further confusion and the need for correction of misleading articles that appeared in the print and electronic media (Starr, 1994).

One other problem in the initial planning stage was an underestimation of the scale of issues, a problem that grew over time. The initial formulation did not include working groups on mental health services, the Indian Health Service, or academic health centers, for example. These were added during the process, as were external review groups and panels of consumers who had written letters to Mrs. Clinton. Meetings and decisions were also delayed by unforeseen events, such as the illness and death of Mrs. Clinton's father in the spring, concerns over campaign financing, and the awareness that the presence of Mrs. Clinton, not being a government employee, raised the question of whether meetings could be secret if she attended.

THE DEBATE ABOUT THE HEALTH INSURANCE REFORM PLAN AND ITS ULTIMATE FAILURE IN CONGRESS

If the initial design and early implementation of the task force was problematic, what developed over the next 100 days and beyond? Why did the proposal ultimately end in failure, with no portions of health care reform passed in that initial session of Congress following the first Clinton inauguration? Two very different types of issues are important as answers. One of these deals with the substance of the plan and problems and limitations of the plan's proposed approach to reform health care. The second kinds of problems were of process, and in some ways are additional aspects of the issues that were explained in the preceding section about the initial development of the health care reform plan.

Problems with the Plan

Reform of health care is a complex area about which health care experts do not agree. This is as true today as it was at the time of the drafting of the Clinton health plan. Certain basic principles, however, are often agreed upon, especially those that focus on provision of access to health care services for all of the population, whether or not they are currently working. Given the experience of rising health care costs in the 1970s and 1980s, most Americans also agree on the need to consider controlling future health care costs as one part of health care reform. It is not necessary to review the plan in detail (and the plan as released to the public was very detailed, over 1300 pages), as it was never implemented; however, there are some substantive criticisms of the approach that help explain why the Clinton health care reform plan failed. One article has reviewed five areas of public choices that contributed to the decline in public support for the plan (Blendon et al., 1995a). Other criticisms are more fundamental (Navarro, 1994).

One of the biggest issues was how to assure universal coverage and whether to link this to an employer mandate. Related to this issue was whether the plan would initially focus on the needs of the middle class (broadly defined) or on the needs of the disadvantaged. Public support, according to a study by Blendon and colleagues (1995a), was twice as high for requiring employers to contribute to health care premiums for full-time workers as it was for part-time workers. Under the Hawaii model, guaranteed coverage was first provided to workers of 20 hours a week or more in 1974, and only extended coverage to those not working or employed for less than 20 hours in 1989. The public was confused about whether health care coverage was guaranteed (in some way, it was for each person through an alliance, although there were to be competing plans and this was complicated for many to follow).

The second problematic issue was the reliance on competing managed care plans as the principal mechanism. While this was done partially as a cost-containment approach and because it lessened the direct role of government involvement, the whole idea increased the public's fear of too much government. It also increased the public's fear of losing the ability to have their own doctors, because they would be forced into a managed care plan or health maintenance organization (HMO).

Related to these two decisions was the third problematic issue of compulsory health alliances. A main feature of the plan was the creation of these large new government agencies (health alliances) in each state that would pool insurance risks and set budget limits on most health care spending. Under the plan, most people would receive health care from a local alliance. This may have been one of the worst substantive parts of the plan, at least in terms of political strategy, since most Americans never understood the concept or how it linked to cost containment. Instead, it provided a target for fears of big government and confused people because there were no clear existing examples of how this worked.

People believed that considerable savings could come from the current system, but many also believed that some tax increase would be required. When the president proposed to raise no new taxes except for those on cigarettes, Americans doubted the integrity of the plan and the honesty of the president and his advisors. As this issue received more discussion and the notion of reliance on anticipated savings in Medicare became known, people feared that the elderly were being asked to subsidize the uninsured. Support declined, especially among the elderly (Blendon et al., 1995a).

Last, the public believed the plan needed to contain costs, and probably controlling insurance premiums would have been the most politically acceptable and easiest approach to understand. Instead, national limits on spending was the approach. To many people, this raised the specter of rationing, long a "hot-button" term in American society. Trust in government was not high enough to accept that this would not lower quality.

In contrast to this approach, which relied heavily on managed competition, the most liberal critics preferred a single-payor approach (Navarro, 1994). This approach would have been simpler to explain in terms of models in other countries, and had already won support from some in Congress in the version of a Health Security Act bill introduced by Senator Wellstone of Minnesota. But its inclusion scared some sectors of business. Instead, the plan opted for a more moderate but comprehensive approach, yet one that was difficult to explain and for which few existing models could be demonstrated. While most health care experts spoke out in favor of the Clinton plan as an important step in comprehensive reform, the enthusiasm of some single-payor advocates was weak.

Problems with the Process

Several aspects of the process as it developed became problematic. Some of these process problems are details of developing the plan and trying to pass it. Others were the lack of development of public support and a public debate. These issues, along with the problems identified about the content of the plan as described in the previous section, all link to the process of achieving reform. The relatively weak position of the Democrats in their congressional majorities was not thought through carefully. Additionally, another problem that occurred was that the delay in development of a plan provided time for opponents to develop their own ideas and materials, including a sophisticated and effective media campaign against the Clinton plan. All of these are process issues, and many experts agree that no comprehensive legislation in any area is without criticism and controversy, so that the failure to pass legislation often turns more on process failures than content failures. Thus, despite the content flaws in the plan discussed in the previous section, probably the more fatal pitfalls for legislative success were those of process.

Development of the Plan and Support

The Clinton administration did initially have a plan for how to have the legislation passed. It was to be introduced within 100 days and fit into the president's budget so that it could all be passed in one piece, as part of the reconciliation bill process described in an earlier chapter. Senate and House leaders both warned the Clintons of the dangers if legislation did not move quickly, especially in the Senate. As spring arrived, one issue that complicated the health legislation was the growing focus on reducing federal deficits, and the need to use Medicare and Medicaid cuts to meet federal deficit reduction targets, rather than being able to keep those savings to balance other new costs from health care reform. Even more important in changing the strategy of using the budget reconciliation process as a way to pass health care reform was the opposition of Senator Robert Byrd of West Virginia, the powerful chairman of the Senate Appropriations Committee. He had a personal rule against adding anything to a budget reconciliation bill that was not related directly to deficit reduction, and he did not believe that the health care plan belonged in the reconciliation budget bill. Byrd was particularly upset because of the rules that apply during the consideration of a reconciliation bill. It could be debated for only 20 hours before it came to an up or down vote. While this might well have improved the chances of passage of the health care plan, Byrd was a traditionalist in his view of the informing function of the Senate, and his belief that American government was designed to make large-scale policy change difficult. The failure to convince Byrd to add the health care plan to the reconciliation bill may have doomed the reform, and Clinton later even agreed that at this point he should have shifted his strategy from achieving comprehensive reform in one bill to a three-year plan (Johnson and Broder, 1996).

As the task force work moved along, a public campaign was also underway. Hilary Clinton held hearings and meetings in many cities, both with health care providers and with the general public. Magaziner, sometimes joined by the First Lady, met with influential members of Congress and interest group leaders. Despite these attempts to focus the attention of the public on the health care reform process, some experts argue that one of the important flaws in the process was the lack of a real public debate and public consensus over the issues (Blendon et al., 1995a; Yankelovich, 1995). Daniel Yankelovich, a public opinion expert, has argued that both the defeat of the catastrophic coverage plan for the elderly in 1989 and the defeat of the Clinton health care reform plan in 1994 reflect a "massive failure of public deliberation" (Yankelovich, 1995, p. 8). He argues that the nation's leadership class (including leaders of medicine, industry, education, the legal profession, science, religion, and journalism) does not talk effectively with the public. All the groups crafting the health care reform plan were from this leadership class, and average Americans did not understand the plan and what it meant for them. Because of this, Yankelovich argues that public support was lost because opponents found it easy to raise public fears about a plan that people did not understand. In support of this argument, Yankelovich demonstrates that public knowledge about the plan decreased over time. Right after Clinton presented his health address to the nation, only 21 percent of the public said they knew much about it. But, instead of increasing over time, by the next month, these numbers had decreased to 17 percent, and they continued to fall until the time that Congress considered the legislation in August 1994, when only 13 percent of Americans felt they were very well informed about the debate in general (Yankelovich, 1995). If the support of the public helps to push major reforms, the public must understand key aspects—at least enough to form an opinion about a proposed plan.

Government Issues

Movement within the Congress was very slow, but Senate Majority Leader Mitchell had plans to introduce one form of legislation in August 1994, and he hoped that the Senate would be able to compromise and agree with the basic tenets of the bill he introduced, which would cover 30 million more Americans for health insurance over the next six years. Senator Robert Dole, as Republican leader, quickly issued a negative statement on the Mitchell bill. Overall press coverage was positive, however, and Representative Gephardt of Missouri introduced a measure in the House that guaranteed to give every American health insurance by 1999, through either private plans financed largely by employers or a vast expansion of Medicare. The American Association for Retired Persons (AARP) endorsed the somewhat limited Mitchell bill and the more liberal Gephardt bill.

At the same time, a debate was occurring in Congress over the crime bill. Newt Gingrich, one of the Republican leaders in the House, managed to oppose the crime bill, create negative press for Clinton, and block a vote on health reform, which he depicted as an example of liberal big government run amok. Because of the problems with the crime bill, which preceded the health care reform bill on the House agenda, health was not considered before the August vacation in the House. On the Senate side, Kerrey declared his opposition to the Mitchell bill and argued for developing a bipartisan coalition with Senator Chafee of Rhode Island and other Republicans in favor of reform. The real issue, however, was concern about declining public support and that the Democrats could lose the Senate if they pushed the Mitchell bill, or a more liberal bill (Johnson and Broder, 1996). Divisions within the Democratic party also became a problem. A mainstream bill was introduced by Chafee, but Democrats could not agree to support it, nor could many Republicans. Dole, as the leader of the Republicans in the Senate, and Gingrich in the House, were not interested in passing a reform bill of any type, believing that the absence of reform would give them a chance at winning major victories in the 1994 off-year elections. Although the crime bill pulled through in August, health care reform did not, and was postponed until Congress came back from vacation in mid-September. By then, most analysts were already saying that health care reform was dead in that session of Congress. As the mainstream coalition effort headed by Chafee met again, Republicans were mobilizing a filibuster in the Senate. The votes to break the filibuster were not there. At the same time, Gingrich announced that if Clinton continued to push for health care reform it would jeopardize Republican support for the GATT (General Agreement on Tariff and Trade). President Clinton believed the GATT was critical to the U.S. economic position as leader of the Western alliance. Mitchell announced that there were not the votes in the Senate to stop a potential filibuster, and that health care reform was dead. Congress would not debate the issue in the closing days of the session.

Analysis of the Problems with the Process

If Yankelovich is correct that the defeat represented a massive failure of public deliberation and was linked to a lack of public understanding about the plan (or plans, as they changed), what does public opinion data show about overall support for the plan? Blendon and colleagues (1995a) also have reviewed public opinion data and concluded that, within a 12-month period, support for the Clinton plan fell from 71 to 43 percent. While some of this loss of support was attributed to substantive choices, as discussed in the previous section, some is attributed to lack of communication with the public—especially the middle class, who became convinced that the plan benefited the poor more than themselves (and perhaps was part of the reason that some Democratic politicians became convinced that they were going to lose the Senate over health care reform). To make the process more difficult, the general public also distrusted the ability of government to do what is right most of the time, an important change over the attitudes of the public in the 1960s, when Medicare and Medicaid were enacted. Thus, building public support is harder in the 1990s, but no less important, especially for a president in a relatively weak position as regards congressional majorities.

Other criticisms and explanations for failure, based partially on process and partially on content, focus on the whole development process and the presentation of the reform plan by the president. A historian who has reviewed the failure of the Clinton health care reform plan has argued that the entire process used by the Clinton administration allowed comprehensive health care reform to be defined as a purely presidential initiative, and did not allow for either public involvement and discussion of trade-offs or for negotiations with Republicans who supported the general goal but did not want to contribute to the triumph of a new Democratic president (Heclo, 1995). In comparison to President Johnson's success in passing his War on Poverty legislation, including Medicare and Medicaid, President

Clinton's reform also became identified as a test of the president's personal popularity, but without the large congressional majorities that allowed Johnson's legislative successes. (In addition, Clinton did not enjoy the understanding of congressional operations that Johnson had gained from his decades of service in the Senate, as well as his strong personal contacts with senators.)

These process problems were compounded by the media campaign that began against the reform plan. If the plan had been proposed and voted on quickly, this type of media campaign might not have developed. The task force missed not only the 100-day deadline, but many others. Some congressional leaders thought it best to wait until the fall. Leaks of alternative plans started to be published in the press, such as a story in the *New York Times* on May 3, 1993, about possible costs of the program. In May, a session to educate the White House staff about options was leaked to the *Washington Post*. The task force was officially disbanded on May 31, 1993. By then, the president was preoccupied with many other concerns, including controversies over the firing of the White House travel staff and the appointment of Lani Guinier as assistant attorney general for civil rights, and the need to have the budget measures passed in Congress. But the leaks and the delays made it possible for an orchestrated public campaign against the plan to have great impact, especially by the time the major bills about health care reform were actually introduced into Congress in August 1994.

Interest groups—especially the HIAA (Health Insurance Association of America), the trade association for small and medium-sized insurance companies, and PRMA (the Pharmaceutical Research and Manufacturers of America)—were opposed to the Health Care Reform Plan, partially because they believed their financial survival was at stake. The delay on release of the proposal until the fall allowed time for development of the media campaign against the bill. The president did not reveal his plan to a nationally televised audience until September 23, 1993. As released, it was an elaborate, 1364-page document and was one of the most comprehensive domestic policy proposals ever made by an American president.

The release of the plan led to extensive news coverage. Between September 1, 1993, and November 30, 1993, over 2000 newspaper, magazine, and television stories about health care were published or broadcast (Rosenstiel, 1994). Interest group spending and attention to the issue were also huge. Over $60 million was devoted to advertising, much provided by HIAA ($14 million) and PRMA ($20 million) (West, Heith, and Goodwin, 1996). A major portion of these funds went to the "Harry and Louise" campaign that in television ads generally showed a middle-class, young professional couple discussing their fears about the plan and how it would limit their choice of doctors, cost them money, or simply would be too complicated to understand, depending upon the particular version. While both sides presented some ads, groups opposed to the Clinton plan outspent supporters by a 2.2-to-1 ratio (West et al., 1996). Moreover, the opponents had their ads ready first, and in the crucial period from October to December 1993, almost all the paid ads were opposed to the program. Whether people remembered any details from the ads, the overall negative advertising helped to derail the Clinton reform plan, not only through its impact on public opinion but also through altering the impression of news reporters and some Washington political elites.

Not all of the problems of process were due to missteps by the Clinton administration. According to more recent reports, some conservative experts had concluded that successful passage of a Clinton health plan would provide an enormous threat to the success of Republicans in the next congressional and presidential elections. Bill Kristol, who worked for the conservative think tank Project for the Republican Future, argued that congressional Republicans should work to kill, rather than amend, the Clinton plan. He argued that doing so would enhance Republican chances of winning Congress and of becoming the majority party, dovetailing with the views of Newt Gingrich, whose "Contract with America" would become a theme for the 1994 elections (Johnson and Broder, 1996). This position became a reality in the plans of the Senate Republicans, who blocked the discussion of health care bills, as well as in the statements of Gingrich on the House side, and in his ability to first delay the health bill and then link its consideration to defeats in other areas.

THE 1994 CONGRESSIONAL ELECTIONS

The 1994 congressional elections had the potential to be major transforming elections in the United States. Republicans gained a majority in both houses of Congress, taking control of the House of Representatives for the first time in 40 years. Gains were large, with 52 seats added in the House and eight in the Senate. While health care was not the only reason the Democrats did poorly in the election, the defeat of health care reform following the initial burst of enthusiasm after Clinton's election was a factor.

Two key questions are: what role did health care issues play in the voters' choices of candidates? and what messages did voters send the new Congress about health care policies? (Blendon et al., 1995b). Blendon and colleagues (1995b) examined public opinion survey data at the time of the election as well as national Election Day exit surveys. Most voters did not choose a candidate for Congress based on health care or even other national issues. Only 22 percent of voters said that stands on national issues were the most important factors, as contrasted with the candidate's experience, character and ethics, and political party. One common thread was unhappiness over the performance of Congress and lack of trust in government, so that incumbents were more vulnerable than usual.

If voters were asked about concerns with specific issues, health appears more important. In data from Election Day surveys, health care was rated as the number one concern in two of the surveys and tied for fourth in the third. Another question asked voters to name their top priorities for the new Congress. Only two surveys asked this question, and health care was listed as number one in both. If a person voted for the Democratic candidate for the House seat, 53 percent named health care as one of the most important issues, versus only 38 percent of those who had voted for a Republican for a House seat. Similarly, in several surveys conducted shortly after the election, health care was named as the number-one priority for the new Congress (Blendon et al., 1995b).

Fewer of the surveys asked what the new Congress should do concerning health care reform and health policy issues. In one survey that asked about health care reform, one-third of voters said they were less supportive than they had been six months earlier. Even among those who had supported Democratic candidates for Congress, 45 percent thought that Congress, not the president, should take the lead in new initiatives. On a more specific question about how to reform health care, by 1994 a majority of voters (55 percent) believed that it was better to have health insurance systems run by private companies rather than by government, versus a more even split (39 percent preferring private companies and 41 percent preferring the government) in 1993. Voters even split over whether the priority should be guaranteeing universal coverage (38 percent) or making an incremental start (36 percent). Twenty percent did not want Congress to attempt to ensure that more people have health insurance.

People do see some groups as more deserving than others. If health insurance cannot be provided to all groups, voters favor covering children first and then people who are uninsured. About half were willing to pay a modest increase in taxes or health insurance premiums to see some changes made in the health care system. Traditional Social Security and health care programs received wide support. Only 17 percent were willing to see cuts in Social Security or Medicaid as ways to deal with deficits, and even fewer (7 to 8 percent) were willing to see cuts in Medicare and veterans' benefits, versus much higher support for welfare cuts in programs such as food stamps, public housing, and AFDC (Aid to Families with Dependent Children).

A policy of cutting the deficit and cutting social programs did receive attention, however, both before the election and after it as part of the Republicans' approach (espoused by Newt Gingrich) of the Contract with America. This was a 10-point-plan that all House Republicans, both incumbents and challengers, signed. It was a conservative agenda for the future, espousing tax cuts, balanced budgets, welfare reform, term limits, and large government cutbacks. Given this agenda of constraining expenditures and cutting back in many kinds of social programs, including health-related ones, combined with the election victories of the Republicans for the second half of the first Clinton term, the last two years of that first term raised new questions about health issues that are discussed in the following chapter. Additionally, the future of the federal role in health care and the unresolved problems in health care in the United States are explored in the next chapter.

7 THE NEED FOR REFORM: FAILURES OF THE CURRENT SYSTEM AND ISSUES OF THE FUTURE

What happens to the health care system of a country after a major attempt at health care reform has failed? What is likely to happen to the U.S. health care system in the future and what will be the federal role? These are the major concluding questions for this book. In answer, first the small reforms that were enacted after the failure of major health care reform and after the Republicans regained control of both Houses of Congress in 1994 will be reviewed. Also, the health care system is not remaining static. Certain trends and changes are occurring, even though they are not a part of federally led health care reform. These changes, however, will set the stage for the new problems that develop and the new issues that become the challenges to solve the next time major health care reform in the United States is proposed. The second section of this chapter will review those trends, in both the growth of managed care and the changing role of the hospital. The last section will speculate on the issues that need addressing in our health care system and the likelihood that either the federal government will be a major factor in health care reform, or trends and changes will be evolutionary and pushed by the system and its own momentum.

REFORMS ENACTED IN THE SECOND PART OF THE FIRST CLINTON TERM

As the public opinion polls after the election showed, most Americans wanted more modest, incremental reform in health care, probably led more by the Congress and less by the president. The Republican Contract with America did not include issues linked to health care.

Although several of the new Republican chairs of congressional committees did introduce modest health insurance reform bills, no major consideration of health issues began until House and Senate budget committees had to consider budget legislation in 1995. The initial expectations were that little attention would be paid to health care in the next few years, because the Democrats had no majority and were leery of losing more credibility on the issue, and because the issue was not important in the new Republican agenda.

As sometimes happens, other issues forced some portion of health care onto the political agenda. One argument about the budget debates concerned trying to balance the budget. The Republicans proposed a budget balanced in 2002 without a tax increase. To accomplish this, reductions in Medicare and Medicaid were required. One proposal would have taken over $250 billion from Medicare, and reduced its annual growth rate by one-third. Large cuts of over $175 billion in Medicaid were also suggested.

At one point, the president was advised to oppose all cuts in the absence of real health care reform. Democrats looked at the plan and were able to publicize the fact that most Medicare recipients could owe another $1000 a year in co-payments, and that many seniors would be forced into HMOs unless they were willing to pay much higher premiums to stay with their own doctors. Some Republicans urged Clinton to create a bipartisan commission to suggest needed changes in Medicare, much as had been successfully accomplished in 1983 with the Social Security Commission, which had saved Social Security from threatened bankruptcy. In April 1995, a report from the Hospital Insurance Trust Fund portion of Medicare indicated that, beginning in 1996, the fund would start to pay out more benefits than it collected in payroll taxes (Johnson and Broder, 1996). Such warnings had occurred before, and the problem had generally been solved by trimming payment schedules to health care providers and/or increasing the Medicare tax rate or raising the amount of income to which the tax was applied. The Democratic interpretation of the Republican plan was that the Republicans were willing to destroy Medicare. Republicans argued that they were not cutting the program, only reducing the rate of increase in the growth of spending. Clinton ended up agreeing to focus on the budget, and proposed a plan to cut the deficit in 10, rather than seven, years. When pushed, President Clinton conceded that his plan would also call for some savings from Medicare and Medicaid. Although some liberals within the party were unhappy, Clinton's strategy eventually assured that the Republicans could not paint a picture of him as fiscally irresponsible. Instead, Clinton was able to present himself to the public as the defender of the old and the poor in a fiscally responsible manner.

By June 1995, to meet their goals of a balanced budget by 2002, the Republicans had to propose enormous cuts of 20 percent in Medicare and 30 percent in Medicaid. Under the initial Republican proposals, the Medicaid program would no longer have been a guaranteed benefit; instead, states would have been able to make major cuts, leaving only immunization and family planning services as federal mandates. At the same time, the Republicans were proposing a tax cut of $245 billion, making it easy for Democrats to argue that Medicare was being cut to benefit disproportionately wealthier taxpayers. Moreover, to make the cuts more appealing to the elderly, the Republicans talked about switching Medicare from a defined benefits plan, in which everyone was eligible for a similar package of services, to a defined payment system, in which each person received the same amount of money and could use it to find the best possible coverage in the marketplace. This idea bears some similarities to the Clinton health care reform idea of managed competition, in which each person would choose the best health care insurance package with subsidies from the government, but would apply only to Medicare recipients, the age group least likely to be familiar with changing aspects of health care insurance, since some have had basic Medicare benefits for over 20 years. Although these cuts passed the House on an almost strictly party line vote in October 1995, the president was not happy about this type of change, as it would change Medicare greatly and not improve access for other Americans.

The cuts passing the House were not the same as a budget being passed by the House and signed by the president. It became clear by late fall that Gingrich was willing to shut down the federal government if President Clinton did not go along with the Republican proposals. By the end of September 1995, 11 of 13 appropriations bills had not been passed, and issues about possible cuts in Medicare and Medicaid had not been resolved. Government shutdowns occurred, first in mid-November and then again later in December after a new temporary spending bill expired. One major aspect of the budget disagreement involved cuts in Medicare and Medicaid, along with other domestic programs. Although the president and the Republicans moved closer on potential sizes of cuts, Clinton refused to agree to the ending of federal responsibility for Medicaid. Eventually, the government reopened and only modest cuts occurred in Medicare and Medicaid.

Just as with major health care reform in the first session of the Congress under President Clinton, few of the major cutbacks in health care programs pushed by the Republicans were passed in 1995. In 1996, both parties wanted to avoid a repetition of the gridlock that, first, major health care reform and, then, the budget impasse had caused in earlier sessions of Congress. As noted in the listing of legislation in the Appendix, some consensus emerged on important incremental reforms that were possible for 1996, just as some minor pieces of legislation had passed in 1994. A commission to deal with border health issues between the United States and

Mexico was established. A Freedom of Access to Clinic Entrances law was passed to protect and promote the safety of people using abortion clinics, in response to the killings of physicians at several facilities. Also, legislation was passed clarifying the definition of a dietary supplement and setting up standards for the labeling and use of such supplements, all in 1994. Small changes in Medicare and Medicaid were also passed that year.

In the election year of 1996, after the debacle of congressional inaction on the budget in 1995, a few modest reforms and changes did occur in health care, on issues on which a bipartisan coalition could be formed. Some amendments were passed to the Food Safety and Safe Drinking Water Laws. The Health Centers Consolidation Act of 1996 was passed to reauthorize and consolidate four federal health, primary care, and prevention programs. These programs included community health centers, primary health centers, health care for the homeless, and health care for residents of public housing. The legislation will help to provide some health care services to medically underserved, low-income populations, although it is very much an example of piecemeal and incremental reform, not a fundamental change to ways in which these types of services are provided to the majority of poor, low-income people. Similarly, small improvements were part of changes to the Indian Health Care Improvement Act. That act extended demonstration programs for direct billing of Medicare, Medicaid, and third-party payors for Indian health care. Amendments to the Ryan White Care Act set some new definitions of eligible areas and populations to receive these AIDS funds, and modified some of the grievance procedures. Again, this and the Veterans Health Care Eligibility Reform Act of 1996 focused on special populations and fixing aspects of the special care systems. For the Veterans bill, eligibility rules were modified and new facility construction was authorized, including provision for additional care for women veterans.

Several other important amendments were added dealing with mental health and HMO care, and the Health Insurance Portability and Accountability Act of 1996, an act with some important health care reforms was passed. The mental health provision may be more important as a reminder of the importance of mental health than in its immediate changes in the health care delivery system. The mental health provision requires that annual and lifetime caps on mental health benefits be at parity with those for physical illnesses. Some plans have had lifetime maximums of $50,000 for mental illness versus $1 million lifetime for physical illness. Some experts point out that if someone has a severe mental illness, resulting in very high expenditures, it is likely to result in the person's losing work and thus health insurance coverage. Were this to be the typical pattern, the legislation might not help the majority of those with severe mental illness. However, it could help parents and spouses of those who develop mental health problems, and is a first step in a recognition that mental illness needs provision for adequate coverage as does physical illness. Another limitation on the mental health provision is that it does not apply to small businesses with less than 50 employees.

The HMO provision is linked to maternity care, and was a clear reaction to the growth of HMOs, which is discussed in the next section. As a cost-cutting technique, some managed care companies had put into effect policies that forced mothers to leave hospitals with their newborns fairly quickly, generally within 24 hours, but in a few instances as soon as 10 hours after a normal vaginal birth. By the time the federal law (Health Insurance Portability and Accountability Act of 1996) was enacted, 30 states had already enacted provisions similar to the new federal ones that require HMOs to allow mothers to stay in the hospital for up to 48 hours after a normal vaginal delivery and up to 96 hours after a Caesarean delivery. Thus, while the new law may not change the actual care available to many people, it sends an important message to HMOs that, given their growth, enrollees may be so concerned that they generate not only state restrictions, but even federal restrictions. As more people receive care from HMOs, their rules and limitations are more likely to become political issues, with the result that more legislation aimed at providing restraints on managed care companies may occur in the future.

The main portions of the Health Insurance and Portability Act involve ending the hesitation of some people to take new jobs because of loss of health insurance as a result of imposition of preexisting clauses for serious health problems. The bill specifically prohibits employers who offer health coverage from limiting or denying coverage to individuals covered under a group health plan for more than 12 months, for a medical condition that was diagnosed or treated in the previous six months. Once the 12-month limit passes, no new preexisting limit may ever be imposed on people who maintain coverage with no more than a 63-day gap, even if they change jobs or health plans. The legislation also prohibits employers from excluding an employee or dependent from coverage because their specific costs are too high. The legislation guarantees renewability of health coverage to employers and individuals except in the case of fraud or misrepresentation by an employer. The legislation also provides for medical savings accounts as an option for small businesses and the self-employed. This is important reform legislation, and it addresses several of the most important problems for employed individuals with health insurance. While these reforms are modest, they are applicable to most employed people, and they benefit employers (by guaranteeing renewability) and employees. These small, incremental changes that deal with major identified problems (job lock for fear of loss of health insurance due to preexisting conditions) may be one of the trends of the rest of this decade.

GENERAL TRENDS IN HEALTH CARE AFTER THE FAILURE OF HEALTH CARE REFORM

Most of the major problems of the health care system that were discussed in 1992 at the beginning of the debate about major health care reform remain now, in 1997, after the reelection of President Clinton and a Republican-controlled House and Senate in November 1996. Small incremental reforms have been passed, including several focused on specialized groups in the population, but major overall reform or restructuring of the U.S. health care system did not occur, and major problems did not disappear. Access to health care is still a major issue, fears of increased costs abound, and problems in funding of Medicare and Medicaid are real.

What is the message the voters sent with the continuation of divided government for four more years? Many experts believe divided government may lead to a few more of the smaller, incremental reforms (as happened in 1996, as both parties wanted to be able to claim small victories in the health care area as they faced the voters in the election in November). Most do not believe that major federally led changes in health care will occur by the year 2000, with the exception of the issue of the Medicare trust fund (and perhaps some attention to Medicaid). Some experts believe that we are beginning to observe major restructuring led not by federal legislation, but by reaction to the need to cut costs and control growth that is occurring in many sectors of the American economy. Relationships in the health care market are undergoing major changes; competitive market forces are dominating the system. Two important aspects of this restructuring are the growth of HMOs and managed care, and the emergence of new organizational structures among physicians, hospitals, and insurers that is resulting in a redefinition of the role of the hospital (Complexity Defines Relationships, 1996). This section will discuss both of these, as well as some of the current problems concerning Medicare and Medicaid.

Growth of Managed Care

One of the trends in U.S. health care today is the growth of managed care in all parts of the country and all sectors of the population, since many states are switching their Medicaid programs to a managed care model and Medicare is also making HMO options available to their enrollees in most parts of the nation (Halvorson, 1996; Kertesz, 1996). HMO enrollment increased in 1995, surpassing 59 million, or 22.4 percent of the U.S. population (Kertesz, 1996). Terms are not always clear in the HMO–managed care areas, but managed care is broader and covers point of enrollment plans, and preferred provider organizations (PPOs). Using these broader definitions, some sources estimate that two-thirds of households are now enrolled in managed care plans, compared with only 39 percent in 1994

(Jensen, 1996). Numbers of plans also expanded, with 126 new plans beginning operation. Being a successful HMO was not as easy, however, and only 61 percent of HMOs reported operating profits in 1995, down from 88 percent in 1994. Related to this, the operating margins of HMOs fell 2.3 percent during the 1995 time period, mainly because of increased medical costs. As an example of the spread of HMOs across the nation, half the new HMOs were in the East, mid-Atlantic, and South Atlantic regions, areas with lower HMO enrollment in the past (Kertesz, 1996).

Consumer satisfaction with HMOs is not as high as in the past. HMO enrollees who reported being satisfied with their plans dropped from 63.6 percent in 1993 to 58.3 percent in 1994 (Jensen, 1996). Those enrolled in Medicare plans actually showed an increase in satisfaction. Many do believe plans are trying harder, with 20 percent stating that their plan's overall performance has improved in the past 12 months and 80 percent being willing to recommend their plan to family and friends. As an example of less satisfied people, 20 percent say they may switch plans at the next opportunity (Jensen, 1996).

Within the HMO field, managed care mergers are one of the trends, with large groups like FHP International Corporation buying out TakeCare, Inc., and Aetna buying PacifiCare, as big plans continue to buy market share (Havighurst, 1996). Some experts believe that physician-run HMOs will not be able to compete with the ever bigger giants of the industry (Votz and Cochrane, 1996). Staff model HMOs are selling their provider groups, as FHP did in selling its physician group and several hospitals recently. How this will affect quality of care and consumer satisfaction is still unclear.

How do these trends of enrollment and satisfaction link to overall assessments of the importance of HMOs as a means by which the private market and competition is restructuring health care delivery within the United States for the rest of this decade? Many experts agree that "health policy in the United States is increasingly focusing, either by design or by default, on managed care as a means of controlling costs" (Luft and Greenlick, 1996, p. 445). While, at their best, HMOs can push preventive care and apply a population-based epidemiological approach to determination of use of health care, much of the literature on the benefits applies only to older group-model HMOs, not the newer forms of managed care (Luft and Greenlick, 1996; Thompson, 1996). It is unclear to what extent many of the cost savings of HMOs were linked to specific historical and environmental factors and may not apply to newer ones developed with less sharply defined models in different kinds of health care environments. While the older-style group and staff model HMOs have delivered good quality care at reasonable cost, the application of this to looser PPO networks and point of service plans is especially unclear (Luft and Greenlick, 1996).

Connected to this issue is the growth of concern by the public about limitations on care, denied hospital and other coverages, and restrictions placed on physicians. Federal legislation has already been passed to restore the option of in-hospital stays for normal deliveries. Other flash points of consumer concern with HMOs are about gag rules for physicians and restrictions on hospitalization for breast cancer surgery (McIlrath, 1996). A proposal to ban gag rules (rules that limit what physicians are allowed to tell their patients in HMOs about alternative treatments not typically supported by the HMO) may be introduced in Congress in 1997. A rash of criticism in late 1996 brought wide attention to the actions by several HMOs to eliminate hospital stays following breast surgery (mastectomies), and the HMO industry hopes to fend off more legislation on this by imposing its own rules (McIlrath, 1996). Recent books by journalists have stressed the concerns about quality of care in HMOs and argued that managed care works only for people who need routine care and checkups, not those with serious or chronic illnesses (Anders, 1996). It is ironic that the fears some Americans had of the proposed Clinton health plan (forcing consumers into alliances and HMO models, severing the preexisting relationships between patients and doctors) are now occurring as part of the growth of managed care. Further trends link to other new organizational structures discussed in the next section.

Emergence of New Organizational Structures and Changes in the Roles of Hospitals

Managed care links to managed competition, which is linked to the idea that, within each market, networks with different and distinct organizational cultures and internal cultures would form and compete, initially on price and style of care and later on quality and value (Complexity Defines Relationships, 1996). While managed competition as the linchpin of reform in the Clinton plan was not enacted, managed competition is becoming the new organizational structure of the future, including major questioning of the role of the hospital in the new health care system. But this is not government-driven and guaranteed managed competition, but rather the workings of the marketplace. In the real world of health care delivery today, some of the best assumptions of managed competition (that consumers would be able to recognize the differences between plans and make plan selections based on comparative value) may not hold. Some experts argue that the structure of the market does not encourage consumer choice because of the paucity of purchasing coalitions for small employers and the lack of standardized benefits, as well as the lack of options that employers provide to employees (Complexity Defines Relationships, 1996). While reengineering is discussed within health care, downsizing does not appear to produce increases in health care and its productivity in the same way that it has in different industrial sectors.

Beyond the growth of managed care for consumers, what is to be the shape of this new competition-driven health care system? One important issue is where hospitals fit into the new care models (Cassil, 1996; Shortell et al., 1995; Stoeckle, 1995; Robinson, 1994). Most observers agree that the acute-care hospital is undergoing a process of rapid, fundamental change. While the hospital has been the central institution of health care delivery (or the "citadel" in Stoeckle's [1995] terminology), this role is being challenged. Hospital occupancy rates are down in most parts of the country, hospitals are not staffing their facilities to serve the maximum number of beds, and most facilities are diversifying into ambulatory diagnostic and surgery centers. Just in terms of numbers, the hospital is an institution on the decline. Because of hospital industry consolidation, the American Hospital Association membership is declining, from 4,694 in 1993 to 4,433 in 1996 (Burda, 1996).

Several articles see new directions as the best approach to survival for traditional inpatient-oriented hospitals. Stoeckle (1995) argues that two general directions are likely. Hospitals can continue to strive for a different expansion of the domain, gaining more diversification and adding a variety of ambulatory care services under the central corporate organization. In this scenario, the central administrative push will be to keep as many beds as possible open. The other direction will be for the hospital to decentralize, affiliate, and redefine itself with new organizations and new practice plans for the community. In this approach, the hospital will not be the center, but will be an adjoining participating institution available for the acute and seriously disabled. Shortell and colleagues (1995) argue that a reinvention process will be necessary for the community hospital, and that it will be to make itself more invisible, hidden within the context of an integrated health system operating as part of a community care network. In slightly differing ways, both of these approaches argue for more complex models of care, ones in which employers may play crucial roles as the major purchasers. Some experts have argued that groups representing the concerns of large purchasers will have to work to see that plans, hospitals, and physicians do not become too focused on being the lowest-cost provider of services, but instead differentiate themselves on the basis of values (Complexity Defines Relationships, 1996). This fits with the essential tenets of managed competition, such as a primary reliance on competition among insurance providers to promote quality care and control costs, with regulation used to prohibit insurers from denying coverage on the basis of health or employment status (Lucas, 1996). In the most optimistic models, long-term care needs could even be met with prefunding by requiring the elderly to purchase long-term care insurance from one among a number of different providers, thus helping to resolve one of the major current problems in the U.S. health care delivery system.

Were these new managed competition models pushed by the market-place, not government reform, to become the norm, the U.S. system would move away in some ways from its traditional dispersed approach to delivery of health care services. It would not, however, fit the more rationalized regional care models discussed at the beginning of this book, since it is not clear how decisions to regionalize care would be made. Different managed care systems (many for-profit and operating in some parts of the country and some metropolitan areas but not others) would make decisions about the spread of new technology. In any given city or region, duplication might still occur, while in other cities needed resources might be absent. A managed competition model would be different from the old, dispersed system (Grumbach and Bodenheimer, 1995). Whether it would be better for more people, provide less expensive care at high quality, and rationalize distribution of expensive health care resources is not clear.

Some trends now do point in the direction of experimentation with this approach for the rest of this decade. Beyond the growth of managed care and the changes in hospitals, some of the recent legislation that reformed Medigap policies in 1990 and the portability legislation of 1996, as well as the requirements that forced HMOs to be more responsive to consumer demand in the area of maternity coverage, are ways to try to ensure that the marketplace provides better information and smoothes its rough edges, while remaining a private-market, competitive approach to delivery of heath care services. A different reading of the years since the failure of health care reform, however, could be that the restructuring is ignoring the concerns of consumers (as with the maternity debate and the concern about outpatient mastectomies). Opposition to new forms of care delivery and rising costs, even as quality and access concerns grow, may lead to more discontent and pressures for more federal intervention and more major health care reform by shortly after the year 2000. Both of these differing scenarios could be impacted by one of the current unresolved issues in the health care area—policy surrounding the current major federal programs, Medicare and Medicaid.

Several different health policy experts have argued that the current situation provides special contradictions. Employers of all sizes have reduced the number of alternative health care plans available to their workers. Traditional fee-for-service medicine is on the decline—now as a result of pushes from the marketplace, rather than pushes from government. One health policy expert argues that "what we're getting is managed care but without the consumer protection and patients' rights that people have a right to expect" (Starr, as quoted in Toner, 1996). Drew Altman, president of the Kaiser Foundation, states "there are a lot of people out there who feel, or should feel, that they fought off the government monster only to find themselves faced with changes in the marketplace that they care about a lot more" (Altman, as quoted in Toner, 1996). Where do these trends leave government, and what is its role in the future U.S. health care delivery system?

Medicare and Medicaid

As the review of legislation since 1965 has demonstrated, many years have contained at least some modifications of the Medicare and Medicaid programs. As much as some experts believe that the next half-decade or decade will focus on nongovernmental actions, some pressures from within the federal government will also drive health care policy. One unrelenting push for government consideration is the Medicare program. Medicare finances health care now for 38 million elderly or disabled Americans, and the trust fund that pays for hospital care, financed out of a fixed payroll tax, will run out of money in the next few years if no further changes in the program occur. The physician trust fund is set up differently, and has unlimited access to the federal Treasury's general revenue, as well as receiving funds from Medicare recipients in the form of premiums paid each month. Medicare is not only large but has become central to budget negotiations over the last decade because it is growing faster than other parts of government. Something will have to occur, and fixing Medicare is likely to be a major topic of debate even within the second term of the Clinton administration.

One of the short-term ways to deal with the program is to cut Medicare spending, such as one proposal by Clinton to cut $138 million over the next six years. To do this, premiums that Medicare pays to health maintenance organizations would be cut, perhaps reducing the viability of some of these plans and penalizing them for efficiency in care. A federal advisory panel has recommended that Congress freeze Medicare payments to hospitals in the 1997 fiscal year, the first time in the history of the program that hospitals would not receive an increase. While in the short run the recommendation of the Prospective Payment Assessment Commission may offer a relatively easy way to reduce the federal deficit and shore up the Medicare Trust Fund, hospitals and integrated health care systems argue that they are being punished for improving their productivity and that this type of short-term fix will not deal with major issues of the future. Some academic health centers that are more dependent on Medicare funds argue they may be placed at special risk, and that these types of cuts will jeopardize the U.S. leadership in health technology.

One other Clinton recommended change is to transfer $60 billion of the costs for home health care out of the Medicare hospital trust fund and into the trust fund that pays doctor bills. Republicans contend this is merely a sleight-of-hand trick to stave off the most immediate crisis in the Medicare hospital fund, but one that increases total health care costs in the overall budget and makes aspects of a budget agreement more difficult in future years.

Medicaid presents other complex issues, especially with the welfare reform legislation passed in 1996. Some see that legislation as the first wave of a movement called "devolution" or "new Federalism" that provides states with more flexibility in how welfare-related programs work and how much they are funded. Clinton was able to preserve most of the Medicaid program as a federal guarantee in 1996; however, some experts predict that the Republicans will call for deeper tax cuts (Stevenson, 1997; Verhoven, 1997). How welfare reforms will actually impact numbers of people on welfare is not clear, and large changes could impact Medicaid in the future.

HEALTH REFORM FOR THE TWENTY-FIRST CENTURY

The twenty-first century is fairly close. Attempts at major restructuring of the U.S. health care delivery system based on federal changes failed in 1994. What will be the defining issues of the future? How does the government and the way it functions make major changes more or less likely? The previous section has reviewed some of the current trends in managed care and competition, the formation of integrated systems of care, and immediate Medicare problems. None of these trends or solutions to the Medicare trust fund issue will resolve one of the major concerns that began the health care reform debate in 1992—problems in access to care. Whether these trends will even hold down rising costs in health care is unclear, and, in Medicare, the aging of the population and the growth in the number of the elderly insured by Medicare will represent a major pressure point on the health care delivery system, even if some short-term reforms in Medicare financing occur. Some of those reforms (limitations on payments to hospitals and HMOs) may cause financial and thus perhaps quality problems in the newly emerging managed competition approach. As previously discussed, pushes to hold down costs by limiting hospital stays for deliveries and breast surgery have led to public outcries and discussions of new federal legislation.

One recent article argues that the five most likely areas of change in the 105th Congress will be: health care coverage, taxation as it relates to Employee Retirement and Income Security Act (ERISA) policy, Medicaid, Medicare, and managed care. Based on a series of informal, semistructured interviews with 16 senior congressional staff and Clinton administration officials, Budetti (1997) concludes that the political chemistry may be too rancorous to permit passage of significant legislation in the near future. Even if this pessimistic assessment is correct, it is helpful to review some of his and his interviewees' conclusions about each of the five areas.

In health care coverage, both the involved policy participants to whom Budetti (1997) spoke and the recent president of the American Public Health Association, at a public session at the 1996 national meeting on access, argue that one likely expansion would be a program that would cover children, perhaps following a Medicare model (Brown, 1996). However, if the current Medicaid program remains protected (as it was by

President Clinton, with his vetoes in 1995 of increased proposed Republican budget cuts), the entitlement for coverage of children below the poverty level up to the age of 19 will be fully implemented by the year 2001, thus possibly mitigating any push for coverage of all children. Other groups of potential policy interest are the unemployed and early retirees. The unemployed are a visible group for policy concern. Similarly, early retirees are a sympathetic and politically active group, especially if retirement is a forced early move due to structural changes in the economy.

On tax and ERISA policy, one possibility is further expansion of medical savings accounts. If ERISA is changed, Congress might permit states to enact mandates requiring employers to provide health insurance coverage (now allowed only for Hawaii). Large, multistate employers would probably lobby against such changes, since they could increase the complexity of benefits negotiations with workers in different states. Major companies prefer to offer similar benefits across different national locations.

Medicaid was a topic of major political debate in the 104th Congress. Republicans proposed reductions in future growth rates and substitution of block grants to the states to replace the federal entitlement to care. However, further push on these seems unlikely at the moment. Medicaid spending rates have slowed, and welfare reform may continue this trend, lowering pressure to reduce growth rates. Because states are beginning to face the reality of fixed budgets for welfare, the interest from the state level in reduced budgets for Medicaid appears to be declining. Some changes may occur, but of a more technical nature, such as a reduction in the payment to federally qualified health centers (they currently receive 100 percent of their reasonable costs rather than having to accept state-determined payment rates). If any cuts come soon, there might be a reduction in the disproportionate-share hospital payment.

In contrast, Medicare has serious financial issues facing it, most of which have already been reviewed in this chapter. Pushes are likely to resolve both spending levels and the future insolvency of the Medicare Part A Trust Fund. In addition to the suggestions mentioned already, Budetti's contacts suggest some interest in a movement to more managed care participation as one solution. These will be shorter-term fixes, however, with solutions of the long-term problem less likely in the next two to four years.

On managed care, Budetti's contacts view the honeymoon period as over, with growing consumer concerns about quality of care and doubts over the long-term cost savings. Even though the Republican majority in Congress is ideologically opposed to mandated benefits and federal regulation of private industry, these types of constraints were passed in 1996 for maternity coverage and are possible in other areas—such as the gag rule for physicians and concern about access to emergency care.

In Budetti's article (1997), the experts see major actions by Congress as unlikely except in the area of Medicare. Some wonder if shared governance and a continued divided government could lessen the overt level of political rhetoric and allow some reform. This analysis would argue that if both parties have some power, they are each vested in the process (Budetti, 1997). Perhaps this is one way around what Steinmo and Watts (1995) identified as the major reason why health care reform in the United States always fails—the bias in political institutions in this country against large reform. This would fit with some of Peterson's (1993) approach, that coalition in support of reform is necessary for major changes to occur. The United States has always been a country in which incremental, rather than major, reform is the usual approach to changing policy. This is true in many areas, not only health care. The election year of 1996 saw some incremental reform, and more may follow. Whether these incremental changes will be enough to gradually improve the system and eventually guarantee a more rational organization with access for all, or whether pressure will build as a result of increased access problems and renewed calls for major health care reform sometime in the early part of the next century, is too difficult to predict. The history of the United States argues against major large-scale reform, but at some point problems may again surface if incremental reform is not able to address the fundamental concerns of access, quality, and cost.

APPENDIX

Selected Federal Legislation with Important Health Aspects (in chronological order)

Merchant Marine Services Act of 1798: Provided health services to U.S. seamen by taxing the employers of merchant seamen; funded the arrangements for their health care through the Marine Hospital Service.

Marine Hospitals Services Act of 1870: Provided a national agency with central headquarters to oversee merchant marine hospitals and staffing.

Federal Quarantine Act of 1878 and Amendments: Gave the Marine Hospital Service the authority to develop quarantine laws for ports that lacked state or local regulation; was expanded to give the service full responsibility for foreign and interstate commerce.

General Immigration Laws of 1882: While this legislation was primarily focused on immigration and not health issues, it included the first medical excludability provisions affecting those who wished to immigrate to the United States. It authorized state officials to board arriving ships to examine the condition of passengers.

Amendment to the General Immigration Laws of 1891: Added the phrase "persons suffering from a loathsome or contagious disease" to the list of medical excludability criteria for immigration into the United States.

Commission Corps Act of 1899 and Amendments: Hired physicians and health personnel to provide public health services.

Biologics Control Act of 1902: Gave the Public Health Service (PHS) the responsibility to license and regulate biologically derived health products.

Public Health and Marine Service Act of 1902: Legitimized the overall coordinating role of the federal government in public health by establishing a communication system for state and territorial health officers.

Pure Food and Drug Act of 1906 (Wiley Act): Allowed the Bureau of Chemistry in the Department of Agriculture to prohibit shipment of impure foods and drugs across state lines.

Vocational Educational Act of 1917 (Smith-Hughes Act): Provided funds to establish early licensed practical nursing (LPN) programs.

The Snyder Act of 1920: The first federal legislation to deal with health care for Native Americans; act provided general assistance and directed the Bureau of Indian Affairs to direct, supervise, and expend monies for the benefit, care, and assistance of Indians throughout the United States.

Maternity and Infancy Act of 1921 (Sheppard-Towner Act): Provided grants to states to plan maternal and child health services; law was allowed to lapse in 1929, although it has served as a prototype for federal grants-in-aid to the states.

Ransdell Act of 1930: Created the National Institute of Health from the Hygienic Laboratory.

Social Security Act of 1935, Including Title V of the Act: Provided for a system of old-age pensions and other old-age benefits, was landmark legislation passed partially as a reaction to the Great Depression; besides the overall establishment of the old-age pension system, Title V included grants to states for maternal and child health and child welfare services, and for services to crippled children; also provided incentives for the establishment of state unemployment funds; Title VI authorized annual federal grants to states for investigation of the problems of disease and sanitation, leading to the creation of new local health departments and significantly increasing overall federal assistance for state and local public health programs.

Walsh-Healy Act of 1936: Authorized federal regulation of industrial safety in companies that were conducting business with the U.S. government.

Federal Food, Drug, and Cosmetic Act of 1938 and Amendments: Regulated market entry of new drug, cosmetic, and therapeutic products for safety by extending federal authority to ban new drugs from the market until they were approved by the Food and Drug Administration (FDA).

Venereal Disease Control Act of 1938 (LaFollette-Bulwinkle Act): Coordinated state efforts to combat syphilis and gonorrhea by providing grants-in-aid to the states to support their investigation and control of venereal disease.

The Reorganization Act of 1939: Transferred the PHS from the Treasury Department to the new Federal Security Agency (FSA). This was changed again in 1953 with the creation of the Department of Health, Education, and Welfare (DHEW) and in 1980 with the creation of the Department of Health and Human Services (DHHS).

The Nurse Training Act of 1941: Provided schools of nursing with support to permit them to increase enrollments and improve their physical facilities.

Public Health Service Act of 1944: Specified a role for the PHS in working with state and local health departments; revised and consolidated into one place all existing legislation pertaining to the U.S. Public Health Service; the legislation provided for the organization, staffing, and functions and activities of the PHS; incorporated the provisions of the Biologics Control Act as a PHS responsibility; allowed use of quarantines and inspections for the control of communicable diseases; also extended services to inmates of penal and correctional institutions; has subsequently been used as a vehicle, through amendments to the legislation, for a number of important federal grant-in-aid programs.

McCarran-Fergurson Act of 1945: Exempted the business of insurance from federal antitrust legislation (such as the Sherman Antitrust Act of 1890 and the Clayton Act of 1914); provided instead that insurance was regulated by state law and did not involve acts of boycott, coercion, or intimidation as the reason why insurance, including health insurance, was exempted.

U.S. National Health Policy Hospital Survey and Construction Act of 1946 (Hill-Burton Amendments to the Public Health Service Act): Provided grants to states to inventory and survey existing hospital and public health care facilities and to plan for new ones; authorized grants to both survey existing facilities and plan construction of new facilities, as well as grants to assist in such construction; required the establishment of state planning agencies and submission of a state plan for the construction of hospital facilities to receive the federal funds.

National Mental Health Act of 1946 (Amendment to the Public Health Service Act): Authorized federal support for mental health research and treatment programs, authorized grants-in-aid to the states for mental health activities; transformed the Division of Mental Health in the PHS into the National Institute of Mental Health.

National Health Act of 1948: Expanded the capacity of NIH by making it the National Institutes of Health and creating a second categorical institute, the National Heart Institute, to go along with the National Cancer Institute.

Water Pollution Control Act of 1948: Partially enacted to deal with benefits to the public health and welfare in abatement of stream pollution; act left the primary responsibility for water pollution control with the states.

Immigration and Nationality Act of 1952 (McCarran-Walter Act): Made major modifications in the immigration laws of the United States, including quotas on countries of origin; primary health issues addressed were modifications in the medical excludability scheme for those wishing to immigrate into the United States.

Medical Facilities Survey and Construction Act of 1954: These amendments to the Hill-Burton Act of 1946 greatly expanded the program's scope by authorizing grants for surveys and construction of diagnostic and treatment centers including hospital outpatient departments, chronic disease hospitals, rehabilitation facilities, and nursing homes.

Air Pollution Control Act of 1955: Provided for a program of research and technical assistance related to air pollution control, justifying the need to deal with air pollution because it represented a danger to the public health and welfare.

Polio Vaccination Assistance Act of 1955: Provided for federal assistance to states for the operation of their polio vaccination program.

Water Pollution Control Act of 1956: These amendments to the Water Pollution Control Act of 1948 created regulatory programs, technical services, and financial aid to the states to assist in their efforts to combat water pollution; urged states to set standards for clean water.

Health Amendments Act of 1956: This amendment to the basic Public Health Service Act of 1944 added special projects dealing with problems of state mental hospitals; also authorized federal assistance for the education and training of health personnel, including traineeships for public health personnel and for the advanced training of nurses.

Dependents Medical Care Act of 1956: Established the Civilian Health and Medical Program of the Uniformed Services (CHAMPUS) for the dependents of military personnel.

National Health Survey Act of 1956: Provided for the first system of regularly collected health-related data by the PHS through the establishment of the Health Interview Survey (HIS) that provides a national household interview study of illness, disability, and health services utilization of the U.S. population.

Amendments of 1958 to Public Health Service Act (PL 85-544): Established a program of formula grants to schools of public health.

Food Additives Amendment of 1958: Amended the Food, Drug, and Cosmetic Act of 1938 to require premarketing clearance from the FDA for new food additives; included the Delaney clause, named after Representative James Delaney, stating that no additive shall be deemed to be safe if it is found to induce cancer when injested by man or animal.

Indian Sanitation Facilities Act of 1959: Provided that the surgeon general construct, improve, extend, or otherwise provide and maintain essential sanitation facilities for Indian homes, communities, and land.

Federal Employees Health Benefit Act of 1959: Permitted Blue Cross to negotiate a contract with the Civil Service Commission to provide health insurance coverage for federal employees.

Social Security Amendments of 1960 (Kerr-Mills Act): Amended the Social Security Act to establish a program of medical assistance for the aged; this program provided aid to the states for payments for medical care for "medically indigent" persons who were 65 years of age or older; state participation was optional, with only 25 states participating; Kerr-Mills program was the forerunner of the Medicaid program established in 1965.

Community Health Services and Facilities Act of 1961: Although passed as a separate statute, this act mostly amended the Hill-Burton Act of 1946 by increasing the amounts of funds available for nursing home construction and by extending the research and demonstration grant program to other medical facilities.

Health Services for Agricultural Migratory Workers Act of 1962 (Amendment to the Public Health Service Act): Established a program of federal grants for family clinics and other health services for migrant workers and their families.

Drug Amendments of 1962 (Kefauver-Harris Amendments): Amended the Food, Drug, and Cosmetic Act of 1938 to strengthen significantly the provisions related to the regulation of therapeutic drugs; required improved manufacturing processes and procedures; also required evidence that new drugs proposed for marketing be effective as well as safe; the amendments followed widespread negative publicity about the serious negative side effects of the drug thalidomide.

Maternal and Child Health and Mental Retardation Planning Amendments; Amendments to Title V of the Social Security Act in 1963, 1965, and 1967: Amended the basic Social Security Act to assist states and communities in preventing and combatting mental retardation through expansion and improvement of the maternal and child and crippled children's programs; added special project grants for maternity and infant care for low-income mothers and infants; added special project grants for child dental services.

Clean Air Act of 1963 and Subsequent Amendments in 1965, 1966, 1967, and 1969: Urged states to set standards for clean air; established cooperative planning with states to set regulations to limit particulate pollution; authorized direct grants to states and local agencies to assist in their air pollution control efforts.

Health Professions Education Assistance Act of 1963 (Amendment to the Public Health Service Act): Provided construction grants for facilities that train physicians, nurses, dentists, podiatrists, pharmacists, and public health personnel; also provided for student loan and scholarship funds to schools of medicine and osteopathy; construction grants were made contingent upon schools increasing their first-year enrollments; later amendments extended loan funds to a variety of health and allied health professions.

Mental Retardation Facilities and Community Mental Health Centers Construction Act of 1963 (Amendment to the Public Health Service Act): Provided construction grants for community mental health centers and for centers for the mentally retarded; facilitates programs to train teachers of mentally retarded, deaf, and other handicapped children; authorized special project grants for training and surveys in community mental health; revised extensively for community mental health programs in 1980, including provisions for comprehensive state mental health systems.

Nurse Training Act of 1964 (Amendment to Public Health Service Act): Added a new title, VIII, to the Public Health Service Act; authorized separate funding for construction grants for schools of nursing, including associate degree and diploma programs; established student loan funds and project grants at schools of nursing.

Hospital and Medical Facilities Amendments of 1964: Amended the Hill-Burton Legislation to earmark grants for modernizing or replacing existing hospitals.

Economic Opportunity Act of 1964 (Also Known as the Antipoverty Program): Mobilized human and financial resources of the nation to combat poverty; various effects on health as it sought ways to improve the economic and social conditions under which many people lived.

Federal Water Pollution Control Act Amendments of 1965 and 1972 Amendments: Switched enforcement responsibilities for water control from the Department of Interior to DHEW and required states to set standards for water quality; 1972 amendments set national rather than state standards for both water quality and sewage treatment; subsequent amendments strengthened the standards.

Heart Disease, Cancer, and Stroke Amendments of 1965 to the Public Health Service Act (Regional Medical Program): Established regional cooperative programs among medical schools, hospitals, and other research institutions; fostered research, training, continuing education and demonstrations of patient care practices related to heart disease, cancer, and stroke.

Health Professions Educational Assistance Amendments of 1965 (Amended the 1963 Act): Authorized basic improvement (institutional grants), special improvement grants, and scholarship grants to schools of medicine, dentistry, osteopathy, optometry, and podiatry; authorized scholarship grants to schools of pharmacy; expanded student loan program and included a provision through which 50 percent of a professional student's loan could be forgiven in exchange for practice in a designated shortage area.

Health Insurance for the Aged of 1965—Title XVIII of the Social Security Act (Medicare) and Amendments: Established a program of national health insurance for the elderly; Part A provided basic protection against the costs of hospital and selected posthospital services; Part B was a voluntary program financed by premium payments from enrollees with matching federal revenues, and provided supplemental medical insurance benefits; amendments added patients who received cash payments under the disability provisions of the Social Security Act through the provision of health insurance for the aged with federal funds; becomes the mechanism for later federal regulations dealing with quality assurance, institutional minimum care standards, utilization review, and cost controls.

Grants to the States for Medical Assistance Programs of 1965—Title XIX of the Social Security Act (Medicaid) and Amendments: Created a federal-state matching program with voluntary state participation to partially replace the Kerr-Mills program; participating states had to provide five basic services: inpatient and outpatient, other laboratory and X-ray, physician, and skilled nursing home services; states could include a number of other optional services; required and optional services changed with amendments; federal categorical welfare recipients were eligible; by option, states could include medically needy with incomes too high for cash federal welfare payments through the provision of health services for low-income federal public assistance recipients and the medically needy; becomes a mechanism for federal regulation of quality assurance, institutional minimum care standards, utilization review, and cost controls in health care.

Appalachian Redevelopment Act of 1965: Dealt with the economic, physical, and social development of the Appalachian region; included the establishment of community health centers in this area and training programs for health personnel.

Older Americans Act of 1965: Established an Administration on Aging to administer, through state agencies, programs for the elderly; covered 10 specific objectives for the elderly, including several relating to health.

Federal Cigarette Labelling and Advertising Act: Required that all cigarettes sold in the United States bear on their labels the message "Caution: Cigarette Smoking May Be Hazardous to Your Health."

Comprehensive Health Planning and Public Health Service Amendments of 1966 (Partnership for Health): Provided for the state and local planning through A and B agencies; provided block grants to state health departments for discretionary purposes; sought to create comprehensive planning for health facilities, services, and personnel within the framework of a federal-state-local partnership; Section 314a authorized grants to states for the development of comprehensive state health planning while Section 314b authorized grants to public or nonprofit organizations for developing comprehensive regional, metropolitan area, or other local area plans.

Allied Health Professions Personnel Training Act of 1966 (Amendment to Public Health Service Act): Construction and improvement grants and traineeships for allied health professions; revised student loan program; patterned after the 1963 Health Professions Assistance Act.

Child Nutrition Act of 1966: Established a federal program of support, including research, for child nutrition; authorized the school breakfast program.

Economic Opportunity Act Amendments of 1966 (Amended the Economic Opportunity Act): Established neighborhood health centers located primarily in impoverished sections of cities and rural areas.

Mental Health Amendments of 1967 and Mental Retardation Amendments to the Mental Retardation Facilities and Community Mental Health Centers Construction Act of 1965: Extended the construction grants to community mental health centers to cover acquisition of existing buildings; extended the program of construction grants for university affiliated and community based facilities for the mentally retarded.

Clinical Laboratory Improvement Act of 1967: Amended the Public Health Service Act to provide for the regulation of laboratories involved in interstate commerce by the Centers for Disease Control through processes of licensure, standard setting, and proficiency testing.

Social Security Amendments of 1967: The first of many modifications to the Medicare and Medicaid programs established by the Social Security Amendments of 1965; provided expanded coverage for durable medical equipment for use in the home, podiatrist services, and outpatient physical therapy, and added 60 days of coverage for inpatient hospital care over and above the original coverage for up to 90 days during any spell of illness; modified some payment rules, generally in favor of providers of care; set conditions that had to be met by nursing homes wanting to participate in the Medicare and Medicaid programs as part of a quality control mechanism.

Health Manpower Act of 1968 (Public Health Service Act Amendment): Extended and modified previous health manpower legislation by authorizing formula institutional grants for training all health personnel.

National Environmental Policy Act of 1969: Consolidated programs dealing with air pollution, water pollution, urban and industrial health, and radiological health; established guidelines for environmental controls for projects involving the federal government; included a new mechanism of environmental impact statements before new projects were begun; allowed for citizen participation; established the Council on Environmental Quality.

Federal Coal Mine and Safety Act of 1969: Helped secure and improve the health and safety of coal miners.

Amendments of 1970 and 1977 to the Clean Air Act of 1963: Allowed Environmental Protection Agency (EPA) to set ambient air quality standards, and set emission standards for plants with high pollution potential; set initial deadlines for auto emission standards.

Water Quality Improvement Act of 1970: Established liability for oil spills; increased restrictions on thermal pollution from nuclear power plants; provided training for all people working in operation and maintenance of water treatment facilities; included requirements for cooperation among various agencies dealing with aspects of water pollution.

Comprehensive Drug Abuse Prevention and Control Act of 1970: Provided for special project grants for drug abuse and drug dependence treatment programs and programs related to drug education.

Poison Prevention and Packaging Act of 1970: Required that most drugs be dispensed in containers designed to be difficult for children to open.

Comprehensive Alcohol Abuse and Alcoholism Prevention, Treatment, and Rehabilitation Act of 1970: Established the National Institute of Alcohol Abuse and Alcoholism; provided a separate statutory base for programs and activities relating to alcohol abuse and alcoholism; included a program of aid to states and localities in their efforts to combat alcohol abuse and alcoholism.

Lead-Based Paint Poisoning Prevention Act of 1970: Represented a specific attempt to address the problem of lead-based paint poisoning through a program of grants to the states to aid them in efforts to combat the problem.

Health Training and Improvement Act of 1970 (Public Health Service Act Amendment): Provided institutional grants for new schools of health professions and special project grants for allied health.

Communicable Disease Control Amendments of 1970 (Amendments to the Public Health Service Act of 1944): Reestablished categorical grant programs to control communicable diseases such as tuberculosis, venereal disease, measles, and rubella; renamed the Communicable Disease Control (CDC) the Centers for Disease Control (CDC); broadened concern beyond the communicable diseases to other preventable conditions such as malnutrition.

Family Planning Services and Population Research Act of 1970 (Amendment to the Public Health Service Act): Established an Office of Population Affairs for family planning, under the assistant secretary for Health and Scientific Affairs; added a Title X, Population Research and Voluntary Family Planning Programs to the Public Health Service Act; authorized a range of projects, including training and research grants and contracts to support family planning programs and services except for abortion.

Emergency Health Personnel Act of 1970 (Amendment to the Public Health Service Act): Authorized the secretary of HEW to assign commissioned officers and other health personnel in the PHS to areas in critical need of staffing; provided the statutory basis for the National Health Service Corps, which sent physicians and other health personnel into areas experiencing health personnel shortages in exchange for education loan forgiveness.

Occupational Safety and Health Act of 1970 (OSHA) and Amendments: Created a strong standard-setting authority vested in the secretary of labor to set a minimum level of protection against specified hazards for workers.

Medical Facilities Construction and Modernization Amendments of 1970: Amended the Hill-Burton Act to add loan guarantees for construction and modernization; added a new area of program grants for emergency rooms, communications networks, and transportation systems.

Comprehensive Health Manpower Training Act of 1971 (Public Health Service Act Amendment): Complex series of amendments that replaced institutional grants with a new system of capitation grants in which health professions schools received fixed sums of money for each student enrolled contingent on increasing first-year enrollments; set up project grants and financial distress grants; revised loan and scholarship provisions so that 85 percent of education loans could be canceled by health professionals who practiced in designated shortage areas; established the National Health Manpower Clearinghouse and directed the secretary of DHEW (now DHHS) to make every effort to provide to counties without physicians at least one National Health Service Corps physician.

Environmental Pesticide Control Act of 1972: Required registration of pesticides; gave EPA authority to ban the use of hazardous pesticides.

National Sickle Cell Anemia Control Act and National Cooley's Anemia Control Act of 1972 (Amendments to the Public Health Service): Authorized grants and contracts for screening, treatment, counseling, and information related to these diseases.

Noise Control Act of 1972: Continued government efforts to rid the environment of harmful influences on human health.

Uniformed Health Services Health Professions Revitalization Act of 1972: Established the Uniformed Services University of the Health Sciences, to be operated under the auspices of the U.S. Department of Defense in Bethesda, MD; created the Armed Forces Health Professions Scholarship Program.

Federal Coal Mine Health and Safety Amendments of 1972 to the Federal Coal Mine Health and Safety Act of 1969: Provided financial benefits and other assistance to coal miners who were afflicted with black lung disease.

National School Lunch and Child Nutrition Amendments of 1972 to the Child Nutrition Act of 1966: Amended the 1966 act to add support for the provision of nutritious diets for pregnant and lactating women and for infants and children (the WIC program).

Consumer Product Safety Act of 1972: Created the Consumer Product Safety Commission to develop safety standards for consumer products; administration of existing legislation such as the Hazardous Substances Act and the Flammable Fabrics Act were transferred to the commission.

Social Security Amendments of 1972 to the Social Security Act of 1935 and the Medicare and Medicaid Amendments of 1965: Made significant changes in the Medicare program to try to control growing costs; established PSROs (Professional Standards Review Organizations) that were to monitor both the quality of services provided to Medicare beneficiaries and the medical necessity for the services; limited payment for capital expenditures that had been disapproved by state or local planning agencies; authorized a program of grants and contracts to conduct experiments to achieve increased efficiency and economy in the provision of health services; also increased access to services for certain groups of people (which raised the costs of the program); people who were eligible for cash benefits under the disability provision of the Social Security Act for at least 24 months were made eligible for medical benefits under the program; persons insured under Social Security and their dependents who required hemodialysis or renal transplantation were defined as disabled for the purpose of having them covered under the Medicare program for the costs of treating their ESRD (end-stage renal disease).

Health Maintenance Organization Act of 1973 (Amendment to the Public Health Service Act) and Amendments in 1976, 1978, and 1981: Specified the basic medical services which a health maintenance organization (HMO) had to provide to be eligible for federal funding; specified requirements for a policy-making board and fiscal responsibility for broad population enrollment; mandated that every employer of 25 or more persons offer an HMO option; amendments mitigated the stringency of the original requirements for HMO service provision to be eligible for federal funding.

Emergency Medical Services Systems Act of 1973 (Amendment to the Public Health Service Act): Established grants and contracts available to states and localities for the development and improvement of area emergency medical systems (EMS) and for related planning.

Older Americans Act of 1973: Established the National Clearinghouse for Information on Aging and created the Federal Council on Aging; legislation also authorized funds to establish gerontology centers; provided grants for training and research related to the field of aging.

National Health Planning and Resources Development Act of 1974 (Amendment to the Public Health Services Act PL-93-641): Added two new titles, XV and XVI, to the Public Health Service Act and substantially replaced the programs established under Sections 314a and 314b of the Comprehensive Health Planning Act of 1966, as well as some of the provisions of the Hill-Burton Act of 1946, by creating a system of local and state planning agencies supported through federal funds; designated State Health Planning and Development Agency (SHPDA) and State Health Coordinating Councils (SHCCs); created a network of local Health Systems Agencies (HSAs) to improve the health of area residents, increase accessibility, acceptability, continuity, and quality of health services, and to restrain health cost increases by preventing duplication of health care services and facilities; permitted the states to establish certificate of need (CON) programs to conduct reviews and make recommendations about new health care facilities and services; regulated funds for new capital expenditures and for renovations for health institutions; provided assistance for modernization or construction of inpatient and outpatient facilities; was repealed by Congress in 1986, leaving responsibility for certificate of need programs entirely in the hands of states.

Safe Drinking Water Act of 1974: Set standards for allowable levels of pollutants and chemicals in public drinking water systems; standards to be established by the EPA.

Social Security Amendments of 1974 (or the Social Services Amendments) to the Social Security Act of 1935: Consolidated existing federal-state social service programs into a block grant program that permitted a ceiling on federal matching funds, also provided more flexibility to states in providing certain social services; added a new title, XX, Grants to the States, to the Social Security Act; focused on prevention and remedy of neglect, abuse, or exploitation of children and adults, preservation of families, and avoidance of inappropriate institutional care; provided some protective, foster, and day care services for children and adults as well as some counseling, family planning, and homemaker services.

Child Abuse Prevention and Treatment Act of 1974: Created the National Center for Child Abuse and Neglect and authorized grants for research and demonstration.

Sudden Infant Death Syndrome Act of 1974 (Added Section XI to the Public Health Service Act of 1944): Developed information programs related to this syndrome for the education of both the public and health professionals.

Employment Retirement Income Security Act of 1974 (ERISA): Regulated pension and benefit plans for employees, including a provision that dealt with exemption of certain health benefits plans from other requirements.

Research in Aging Act of 1974: Created the National Institute of Aging as part of the NIH.

Congressional Budget and Impoundment Act of 1974: Established the U.S. Congressional Budget Office (CBO), which conducts studies on the fiscal and budget implications of new laws, including those related to health.

Nonprofit Hospital Amendments of 1974 (Amendment to the Taft-Hartley Act of 1947): Ended the exclusion of nongovernmental nonprofit hospitals from the provision of the Taft-Hartley and the Wagner Acts.

Health Professions Education Assistance Act of 1976 (Amendment to the Public Health Service Act of 1944): Extended capitation and special project grants to schools of public health and health administration programs; broadened start-up grants, special project grants, and construction and traineeship grants; changed capitation grant prerequisites by dropping the requirement that schools increase first-year enrollment and instead emphasized primary care by requiring that medical schools have 50 percent of their graduates enter residency programs in primary care by 1980.

Medical Devices Amendment of 1976 (Amendment to the Federal Food, Drug, and Cosmetic Act of 1944): Strengthened the regulation of medical devices, partially as a reaction to concerns over the Dalkon Shield intrauterine device.

Resource Conservation Recovery Act of 1976 and Amendments: Developed management and review plans for safe disposal of discarded material; regulated management of hazardous wastes.

Toxic Substances Control Act of 1976: Regulated chemical substances affecting health and the environment; provided grants to the states; included the development of a data system for research and regulation; banned the manufacture and use of polychlorinated biphenyls (PCBs).

Health Maintenance Organization Amendments of 1977 (Amended the 1973 Health Maintenance Organization Act): Eased the requirements that had to be met for an HMO to be federally qualified; required that an HMO had to be federally qualified to receive Medicare and Medicaid funds.

Indian Health Care Improvement Act of 1977: A large piece of legislation dealing with filling gaps in the delivery of health care services to Native Americans, mostly through the IHS (Indian Health Service).

National Consumer Health Information and Health Promotion Act of 1977 (Amendment to the Public Health Service Act of 1944): Authorized grants and contracts for research and community programs related to health information, health promotion, preventive health services, and education of the public in the use of appropriate health care services.

Clean Water Act of 1977: Created best (conventional) technology standards for water quality by 1984; raised liability limits on oil spill cleanup costs.

Rural Health Care Services Amendments of 1977 (Amendments to the Medicare and Medicaid Legislation of 1965): Modified the categories of practitioners that could provide services under these programs; rural health clinics that did not routinely have physicians on site could be reimbursed for services provided by nurse practitioners if they met certain requirements; also authorized demonstration projects with these practitioners for underserved urban areas.

Medicare and Medicaid Antifraud and Abuse Amendments of 1977 (Amendments to the Medicare and Medicaid Legislation of 1965): Tried to reduce fraud and abuse in the programs as a means to help contain costs; strengthened criminal and civil penalties for fraud and abuse; modified the operation of PSROs; required uniform reporting systems and formats for hospitals and certain other health care organizations participating in Medicare and Medicaid.

Medicare End-Stage Renal Disease Amendments of 1978 (Further Amendments to the Medicare and Medicaid Legislation of 1965 that Had Been Amended in 1972 to Create the ESRD Program): Changed the program slightly to attempt to control costs by adding incentives to encourage the use of home dialysis and the use of renal transplantation; authorized funding for studies of ESRD treatments.

Health Maintenance Organization Amendments of 1978 (Amended the 1973 Health Maintenance Organization Act): Added a program of loans and loan guarantees to support new ambulatory facilities and related equipment; supported a program to train HMO administrators and medical directors to provide technical assistance to HMOs in their developmental efforts.

Health Planning and Resources Development Amendments of 1979 (Amendments to the 1974 National Health Planning and Resources Development Act): Included provisions to encourage competition within the health care sector; dealt with the need to integrate mental health and alcoholism and drug abuse resources into health system plans.

Comprehensive Environmental Response, Compensation, and Liability Act of 1980: Created federal superfund to clean up chemical dumps and toxic wastes; authorized EPA to sue responsible parties for toxic spills for recovery of government cleanup expenses.

Mental Health Systems Act of 1980 (Amendments to the Community Mental Health Centers Act of 1970): Included extensive changes to the Community Mental Health Systems Program, including provisions for the development and support of comprehensive state mental health systems; legislation was quickly superseded by the block grants to the states for mental health and alcohol and drug abuse treatment that were part of the Omnibus Budget Reconciliation Act of 1981.

Omnibus Budget Reconciliation Act (OBRA) of 1980: Was contained as part of Title IX of Medicare and Medicaid Amendments of 1980; extensive modifications in the Medicare and Medicaid programs aimed at dealing with the growing costs of the programs; some changes in Medicare included the removal of the 100 visits/year limitation on home health services, requirement of a deductible for home care visits under Part B, permission for small rural hospitals to use swing beds (alternate between acute or long-term care beds as the need occurs), and authorization for demonstration programs of swing beds in large urban hospitals; most important change for Medicaid was requiring the program to pay for the services that the states had authorized nurse-midwives to perform.

Omnibus Budget Reconciliation Act (OBRA) of 1981: In Title XXI, Subtitles A, B, and C provided further amendments to the Medicare and Medicaid programs; this legislation also included extensive changes to that program with 46 sections, some including eliminating the coverage of alcohol detoxification facilities, removing occupational therapy as a basis for entitlement for home health services, and increasing the Part B deductible; replaced 20 categorical programs in areas of prevention, alcohol and drug abuse, mental health, primary care, and some areas of maternal and child health with four block grants in the major areas listed above; reduced funds by 25 percent in the process of replacing categorical programs with block grants; in the preventive programs area, consolidated separate programs such as rodent control, fluoridation, hypertension control, and rape crisis centers into one block grant distributed among the states by a formula based on population and other factors; in the mental health area, combined the existing programs (the Community Mental Health Centers Act, the Mental Health Systems Act, the Comprehensive Alcohol Abuse and Alcoholism Prevention, Treatment, and Rehabilitation Act, and the Drug Abuse Prevention, Treatment, and Rehabilitation Act); in the Primary Care Block Grant replaced the Community Health Centers; in the Maternal and Child Health Block Grant consolidated seven categorical programs from Title V of the Social Security Act and the Public Health Service Act, including maternal health and crippled children's programs, SIDS, genetic disease services, hemophilia treatment, SSI payments to disabled children, and lead-based poisoning programs.

Orphan Drug Act of 1982: Provided financial incentives for the development and marketing of orphan drugs, defined by the legislation as drugs for the treatment of diseases or conditions affecting so few people that revenues from the sales of the drugs would not cover their development costs.

Tax Equity and Fiscal Responsibility Act of 1982 (TEFRA): Made important changes in the Medicare and Medicaid programs and in some other health-related programs; replaced PSROs that had been established by the Social Security Amendments of 1972 and eliminated requirements for local HSAs, cut their funding, and increased gubernatorial discretion concerning their future role; replaced PSROs with Professional Review Organizations (PROs) and made their use in hospitals optional for patients covered under government programs; for Medicare, made extensive changes in reimbursement methodologies for hospital-related services under Medicare; began a shift to casemix (diagnostic related groups) for reimbursements for most acute-care hospitals; eliminated nursing salary cost differentials and private room subsidies; eliminated the lesser of cost or charge provision; made reimbursement changes for HMOs; for Medicaid, tightened regulations on acceptable error rates and overpayments and made a number of changes in payment methodology; added coverage for hospice services to Medicare benefits; reduced Medicaid funding for states, but allowed a partial gainback for improved program administration,including fraud detection and error-rate reduction; eliminated capitation payments for nursing and medical schools and reduced capitation payments for selected other health professional schools; greatly reduced funding for new entrants into the National Health Service Corps.

Social Security Amendments of 1983: A major landmark in the Medicare program, this legislation amended the basic rules of the Medicare program to create a prospective payment system for hospital care by basing payments to hospitals on predetermined rates per discharge for diagnosis related groups (DRGs), as contrasted to the earlier cost-based system of reimbursement that had been used since the initial passage of the Medicare Program; began a study of physician payment reform options.

Deficit Reduction Act of 1984 (DEFRA): Temporarily froze increases in physician payment under Medicare; placed a specific limit on the rate of increase in the DRG payment rates in the following two years; established the Medicare Participating Physician and Supplier Program (PAR) that created two classes of physicians in regards to their relationships to the Medicare program, and outlined different reimbursement approaches for them depending upon whether one was classified as "participating" or "nonparticipating"; mandated that the Office of Technology Assessment study alternative means of paying for physicians' services to guide reform of Medicare.

Child Abuse Amendments of 1984 (Amendments to the Child Abuse Prevention and Treatment Act of 1974): Involved infant care review committees in the decision about the treatment of handicapped newborns; established treatment and reporting guidelines for severely disabled newborns.

National Organ Transplant Act of 1984: Made it illegal to acquire, receive, or transfer any human organ for valuable consideration for use in human transplantation if it involved interstate commerce.

Drug Price Competition and Patent Team Restoration Act of 1984: Gave brand-name pharmaceutical manufacturers patent term extensions.

Consolidated Omnibus Budget Reconciliation Act of 1985 (COBRA '85): Especially impacted the Medicare program by adjusting the disproportionate share payments made to hospitals that served many poor patients; hospice care was made a permanent part of Medicare and made available to states also under Medicaid; froze prospective payment system (PPS) payment rates for part of the year; modified hospital indirect rates for medical education; established PPRC (Physician Payment Review Commission) to aid Congress on physician payment policies; required that employers continue health insurance for employees and their dependents who would otherwise lose their eligibility due to reduced hours or termination of employment.

Emergency Deficit Reduction and Balanced Budget Act (Graham-Rudman-Hollins Act) of 1985: Established mandatory deficit reduction targets for five subsequent fiscal years; led to significant impact on the Medicare program in the latter half of the 1980s, and on other health programs also.

Omnibus Budget Reconciliation Act of 1986 (OBRA '86): Altered PPS payment rates for hospitals; reduced payment amounts for capital-related costs; established further limits to balance billing by physicians by setting maximum allowable charges for physicians who did not participate in the PAR program.

Omnibus Health Act of 1986: Liberalized coverage under the Medicaid program by using income up to the federal poverty line as a criterion; allowed states to offer infants up to one year and all pregnant women coverage, with a phase-in schedule for coverage up to five years of age; included the National Childhood Vaccine Injury Act that established a federal vaccine injury compensation program; also included the Health Care Quality Improvement Act that provided immunity from private-damage lawsuits under federal or state law for a professional review action that followed standards set out in the legislation.

State Comprehensive Mental Health Services Plan Act of 1986: Built on the Community Support Program established as a demonstration program by NIMH to authorize each state to work with the Medicaid agency and provide a detailed plan for care of individuals with serious mental illness.

National Health Service Corps Amendments of 1987 (Revision to the Emergency Health Personnel Act of 1970): Reauthorized the National Health Service Corps (NHSC), initially authorized under the 1970 legislation.

Omnibus Budget Reconciliation Act of 1987 (OBRA '87): Altered a number of aspects of both Medicare and Medicaid; for Medicare, the wage index used to calculate hospital payments was updated, and capital-related costs were reduced by 12 percent for fiscal year 1988 and 15 percent for fiscal year 1989; for physician payment, fees for 12 over-valued procedures were reduced and higher fee increases were allowed for primary care than for specialized physician services; for Medicaid, states were required to cover eligible children up to age six with an option for up to age eight; the distinction between skilled nursing facilities and intermediate care facilities was eliminated, and a number of provisions designed to enhance the quality of care in nursing homes were included.

Medical Waste Tracking Act of 1988: In reaction to the concern over the number of used and discarded syringes washing ashore in the eastern United States, the bill focused on improved tracking of medical wastes from their origin to their disposal.

Medicare Catastrophic Coverage Act of 1988 (Amendment to the Medicare Act of 1965): Provided the largest expansion of benefits since the creation of the program; added coverage for outpatient drugs and respite care, and placed a cap on out-of-pocket spending for co-payment costs and covered services; costs were to come from increased premiums to all Medicare enrollees and an income-related supplemental premium; was repealed before provisions went into effect.

National Organ Transplant Amendments of 1988 (Amendments to the National Organ Transplant Act of 1984): Amended the earlier act to extend the prohibition against the sale of human organs to the organs and body parts of human fetuses.

The Technical and Miscellaneous Revenue Act of 1988: Told the PPRC to consider policies to moderate the rate of increase in expenditures for physician services in Medicare programs, and for reducing the utilization of these services.

Omnibus Budget Reconciliation Act of 1989 (OBRA '89): Included provisions for minor, predominantly technical changes in the PPS; extended some coverage for mental health benefits and Pap smears; small adjustments in disproportionate share rules; the major change was to begin the implementation of a resource-based relative value scale (RBRVS) for physician payment, phased in over a four-year period starting with 1992; created the new Agency for Health Care Policy and Research (AHCPR) to replace the National Center for Health Services Research and Technology Assessment (NCHSR); focus of the new agency was to conduct and foster studies of health care quality, effectiveness, and efficiency, including those on outcomes of medical care treatment.

Safe Medical Devices Act of 1990 (Amendments to the Federal Food, Drug, and Cosmetic Act of 1938 and Medical Devices Amendment of 1976): Required institutions that use medical devices to report device-related problems to the manufacturer and to the FDA.

Americans with Disabilities Act (ADA) of 1990: Provided a broad range of protections for the disabled, and thus combined former protections from the Civil Rights Act of 1964, the Rehabilitation Act of 1973, and the Civil Rights Restoration Act of 1988; the legislation helps the disabled toward a goal of independence and self-support.

Immigration and Nationality Act of 1990 (Modification of Immigration and Nationality Act of 1950): Restructured with minor modifications the medical exclusion scheme used to screen people who wish to immigrate to the United States.

Omnibus Budget Reconciliation Act of 1990 (OBRA '90): Included the Patient Self-Determination Act, minor changes in the PPS, and other technical adjustments to payments for Medicare; the Patient Self-Determination Act required health care institutions that participate in Medicare and Medicaid to provide all patients with written information on policies regarding self-determination and living wills, and to inquire whether patients had advance medical directives; further adjustments were made in the PPS wage index calculation, and the capital-related payment reduction; as part of deficit reduction, there was included a five-year deficit reduction plan to reduce Medicare outlays by over $43 billion between fiscal years 1991 and 1995; one important change was to require that all Medigap policies sold after July 1992 had to conform to one of 10 standardized packages so that consumers could more easily compare coverage and costs from one insurance company to another.

Ryan White Comprehensive AIDS Resources Emergency Act of 1990 (Amendment to the Public Health Service Act of 1944): Set up special programs to distribute funds related to AIDS through grants, and created mechanisms to involve the public in the process; created mechanisms for planning and evaluation of the process.

National Institutes of Health Revitalization Act of 1993: Provided for some structural and budgetary changes in the operation of the NIH; also included guidelines for the conduct of research on transplantation of human fetal tissue and added HIV infection to the list of excludable conditions covered by the Immigration and Nationality Act.

Omnibus Budget Reconciliation Act of 1993 (OBRA '93): Put into place a record five-year cut in Medicare funding; included other changes in Medicare such as provision to end return on equity (ROE) payments for capital to proprietary skilled nursing facility (SNFs); reduced the rate of increase of inpatient rates for care provided in hospices; cut laboratory fees and froze payments for durable medical equipment, parenteral and enteral services, and orthotics and prosthetics; included the Comprehensive Childhood Immunization Act to support the provision of vaccines for children eligible for Medicaid, children without health insurance, and Native American children.

Dietary Supplement Health and Education Act of 1994: Clarified the definition of a dietary supplement and set up standards for labeling and proper use of such, including supplemental labelling; set requirements for new dietary ingredients that are supplements.

Freedom of Access to Clinic Entrances Act of 1994: Protected and promoted the public safety and health by establishing federal penalties and civil remedies for certain violent, threatening, and obstructive conduct that interfered with people obtaining reproductive health services; enacted as a response to bombings of abortion clinics and killings of physicians at several of the clinics.

Social Security Act Amendments of 1994: Made a number of technical and other changes in the Medicare program; modified the Maternal and Child Health Block Grant program and income security, human resources, and related programs; for Medicare, adjusted standardized amounts for wages and wage-related costs, provided more coverage for psychologists, refined the geographic cost of practice index for physician payment, limited extra billing of physicians, required the creation of complete relative values for pediatric services as had been earlier done for other types of services, modified durable medical equipment rules, set in place mammography certification requirements, placed an annual cap on Medicare payment for outpatient physical therapy and occupational therapy services, and provided speech-language pathology and audiology services; in maternal and child welfare, increased the authorization and placed more emphasis on protections for foster children, child welfare traineeships, and payments of state claims for foster care and adoption assistance, added new enforcement procedures in child support along with other changes more linked to the welfare side than medical services.

United States–Mexico Border Health Commission Act of 1994: Authorized and encouraged the president to conclude an agreement with Mexico to establish a binational commission to deal with border health issues, including coordination of public health efforts and education of the population about health problems; included provisions for research and studies on the topic.

Veterans Health Programs Extension Act of 1994: Added the treatment of sexual trauma and repealed the time limitation for seeking therapy; increased research relating to women veterans; increased authority to provide priority health care for veterans exposed to toxic substances.

1995 Amendment to Omnibus Budget Reconciliation Act of 1990: Permitted select policies to be offered in all states for an extended period of time.

1995 Amendment to Public Health Service Act of 1944: Permanently extended and clarified malpractice coverage for health centers.

1996 Amendment to the Public Health Service Act of 1944, Part J of Title III: Provided for expanded studies and establishment of innovative programs in the area of traumatic brain injury.

Food Safety Protection Act of 1996 (Replaced the Delaney Clause of the Food, Drug, and Cosmetics Act of 1958): Set new limits on pesticide use in food production, banned any residue of pesticide that causes cancer.

Health Centers Consolidation Act of 1996 (Amendment to the Public Health Service Act of 1944 and Its Amendments): Consolidated and more clearly defined health centers, primary care services, and medically underserved areas; included planning grants and managed care loan guarantees; included special provisions for services to the homeless.

Health Insurance Portability and Accountability Act of 1996 (Also Known as the Kennedy-Kassebaum Act): Improved portability and continuity of health insurance coverage in group and individual markets when an individual loses a job; promoted the use of medical savings accounts, improved access to long-term care services and coverage; stipulated changes in the membership and duties of the national committee on vital and health statistics.

Indian Health Care Improvement Technical Corrections Act of 1996 (Amendment to the Indian Health Care Improvement Act of 1977): Extended demonstration programs for direct billing of Medicare, Medicaid, and other third-party payors.

Ryan White Care Act Amendments of 1996 (Amendments to the Ryan White Comprehensive AIDS Resources Emergency Act of 1990): Set new definitions of eligible areas and eligible population numbers; made modifications in membership of the councils to aid in distribution of funds; modified grievance procedures over grant distribution, and modified some aspects of grant application, planning, and evaluation.

Safe Drinking Water Act Amendments of 1996: Created right-to-know requirements that oblige officials of drinking water systems to tell customers about contamination problems by mail; provided funds to improve water treatment plants and mandated new standards for arsenic, radon, and several other contaminants.

Small Business Job Protection Act of 1996: Included many nonhealth-related provisions but also clarified application of ERISA; recategorized the Orphan Drug Tax Credit as a business credit.

Veterans Health Care Eligibility Reform Act of 1996: Amended previous veterans' health care legislation to reform eligibility for health care provided by the Department of Veterans Affairs, especially so as to provide care to the extent and amount provided in advance by authorization legislation and, as part of this, separate outpatient care priorities from inpatient care priorities were deleted; authorized major facility construction projects for the department and improved administration of health care by the department; provided for more care for women veterans; readjusted counseling and mental health care; authorized special studies on hospice care, special pay arrangements for physicians and dentists who enter residency training, and evaluation of the health status of spouses and children of Persian Gulf War veterans.

REFERENCES

Access to Health Care in the United States: Results of a 1986 Survey. Special Report Number 2. Princeton, NJ: Robert Wood Johnson Foundation, 1987.

Aday, L., R. Andersen, and G. Fleming. *Health Care in the United States: Equitable for Whom?* London: Sage Publications, 1980.

Alford, Robert R. *Health Care Politics: Ideological and Interest Group Barriers to Reform.* Chicago: University of Chicago Press, 1975.

Anders, George. *Health Against Wealth.* Boston: Houghton Mifflin Co., 1996.

Andersen, Ronald M., and Pamela L. Davidson. "Measuring Access and Trends." In *Changing the U.S. Health Care Delivery System,* edited by Ronald M. Andersen, Thomas H. Rice, and Gerald F. Kominski. San Francisco: Jossey-Bass Publishers, 1996.

Anderson, Odin. *Health Care: Can There Be Equity?* New York: Wiley, 1972.

Anderson, Odin, and J.J. Feldman. *Family Medical Costs and Voluntary Health Insurance: A Nationwide Study.* New York: McGraw-Hill, 1956.

A New Survey on Access to Medical Care. Special Report Number 1. Princeton, NJ: Robert Wood Johnson Foundation, 1978.

Angell, M. "How Much Will Health Care Reform Cost?" *New England Journal of Medicine* 328: 1778–1779, June 17, 1993.

Aries, N., and L. Kennedy. "The Health Labor Force: The Effects of Change." In *The Sociology Of Health and Illness: Critical Perspectives,* edited by P. Conrad and R. Kern. New York: St. Martin's Press, 1990.

Barnett, P.G., and J.E. Midling. "Public Policy and the Supply of Primary Care Physicians." *Journal of the American Medical Association* 262: 2864–2868, 1989.

Banta, D., C. Behny, and J. Wilems. *Toward Rational Technology in Medicine.* New York: Singer, 1981.

Bean, Pamela, and Kathryn Waldron. "Readmission Study Leads to Continuum of Care." *Nursing Management* 26: 65–68, 1995.

Bilheimer, Linda T., and Robert D. Reischauer. "Confessions of the Estimators." *Health Affairs* 14: 37–55, 1995.

Blendon, Robert J. "Satisfaction with Health Systems in Ten Nations." *Health Affairs* 9: 185–192, 1990.

Blendon, Robert J., Mollyann Brodie, and John Benson. "What Happened to Americans' Support for the Clinton Health Plan?" *Health Affairs* 14: 7–23, 1995a.

Blendon, Robert J., Drew E. Altman, John Benson, Mollyann Brodie, Matt James, and Gerry Chervinsky. "Health Care Policy Implications of the 1994 Elections." *Journal of the American Medical Association* 273: 671–674, 1995b.

Blendon, Robert J., Karen Donelan, Craig A. Hill, W. Carter, D. Beatrice and Drew Altman. "Paying Medical Bills in the United States: Why Health Insurance Isn't Enough." *Journal of the American Medical Association* 271: 949–951, 1994.

Boland, Peter. "The Role of Reengineering in Healthcare Delivery." *Healthcare Leadership Care* 15: 5, 1996.

Botelho, Richard J. "Overcoming the Prejeudice Against Establishing a National Health Care System." *Caring for the Uninsured and Underinsured*. Chicago: American Medical Association, 1991.

Brown, E. Richard. "Access to Care." Session Featuring the American Public Health Association President. APHA Annual Meeting, Washington, DC, 1996.

Brown, E. Richard, and Roberta Wyn. "Public Policies to Extend Health Care Coverage." In *Changing the U.S. Health Care Delivery System*, edited by Ronald M. Andersen, Thomas H. Rice, and Gerald F. Kominski. San Francisco: Jossey-Bass Publishers, 1996.

Budetti, Peter. "Health Reform for the 21st Century." *Journal of the American Medical Association* 277: 193–198, 1997.

Burda, David. "AHA Buffeted by Industry Changes." *Modern Healthcare*, p. 50, October 7, 1996.

Cascardo, D. "Factors Affecting Cost Containment in an HMO: A Review of the Literature." *Journal of Ambulatory Care Management* 5: 53–63, 1982.

Cassil, Alwyn. "Hospitals Can Expect Anything But Status Quo." *AHA News*, p. 1, November 11, 1996.

Chelf, Carl P. *Public Policymaking in America: Difficult Choices, Limited Solutions*. Santa Monica, CA: Goodyear, 1981.

Christianson, J.B., D.R. Wholey, and S.M. Sanchez. "State Responses to HMO Failures." *Health Affairs* 10: 78–92, 1991.

Cohodes, D.R. "The Home of the Free, the Land of the Uninsured." *Inquiry* 23: 227–235, 1986.

Colwill, J.M. "Where Have All the Primary Care Applicants Gone?" *New England Journal of Medicine* 326: 387–408, 1992.

"Complexity Defines Relationships in Increasingly Competitive Marketplaces." *Health Care Financing and Organization News and Progress*. Washington, DC: Alpha Center, pp. 1–4, November 1996.

Cowan, Cathy A., Bradley R. Braden, Patricia A. McDonnell, and Lekha Sivarajan. "Business, Households and Government: Health Spending, 1994." *Health Care Financing Review* 17: 157–178, 1996.

"Crash: Piecing Together the Continuum of Care." *Hospitals and Health Networks*, pp. 26, 28, November 20, 1994.

Davis, K., M. Gold, and D. Maleac. "Access to Health Care for the Poor." *Annual Review of Public Health* 2: 150–182, 1981.

Dawson, W. "Interim Report on the Future Provision of Medical And Allied Services." In *The Regionalization of Personal Health Services*, edited by E.D. Saward. New York: Prodist, 1975.

Delavan, S.M. and S.Z. Koff. "The Nursery Shortage and Provider Attitudes: A Political Perspective." *Journal of Public Health Policy* 11: 62–80, 1990.

DesHarnais, S., E. Kobrinski, and J. Chesney. "The Early Effects of the PPS on Inpatient Utilization and the Quality of Care." *Inquiry* 24: 7–16, 1987.

Diamond, Martin. *The Founding of the Democratic Republic*. Itasca, IL: F.E. Peacock Publishers, 1981.

Donelan, Karen, Robert J. Blendon, Craig A. Hill, Catherine Hoffmak, Dianne Rowland, Martin Frankel, and Drew Altman. "Whatever Happened to the Health Care Crisis in the United States?" *Journal of the American Medical Association* 276: 1346–1350, 1996.

Drew, Elizabeth. "Politics and Money, Part I." *The New Yorker*, December 6, pp. 54–119, 1982a.

Drew, Elizabeth. "Politics and Money, Part II." *The New Yorker*, December 13, pp. 57–111, 1982b.

Edwards, W.O., and C.R. Fisher. "Medicare Physician and Hospital Utilization and Expenditure Trends." *Health Care Financing Review* 11: 111–116, 1989.

Enthoven, Alain. *Health Plan: The Only Practical Solution to the Soaring Costs of Medical Care*. Reading, MA: Addison-Wesley, 1980.

Estes, Carol C. *The Aging Enterprise*. San Francisco, CA: Jossey-Bass Publishers, 1980.

Evashwick, Connie J. "The Continuum of Care." In *Introduction to Health Services*, 4th ed., edited by Stephen J. Williams and Paul R. Torrens. Albany, NY: Delmar, 1993.

Fein, Rashi. "Social and Economic Attitudes Shaping American Health Policy." *Milbank Memorial Fund Quarterly/Health and Society* 58: 349–385, 1980.

Fraser, I., J. Narcross, and P. Kralovec. "Medicaid Shortfall and Total Unreimbursed Hospital Care for the Poor, 1980–1989." *Inquiry* 28: 385–392, 1991.

Freeman, H.E., R.J. Blendon, L.H. Aiken, S. Sudman, C.F. Mullinix, and C.R. Corey. "Americans Report on Their Access to Health Care." *Health Affairs* 6: 11–27, Spring 1987.

Freidson, Eliot. *Profession of Medicine: A Study of the Sociology of Applied Knowledge*. New York: Dodd, Mead and Co., 1970.

Freidson, Eliot. "The Medical Profession in Transition." In *Applications of Social Science to Clinical Medicine and Health Policy*, edited by L. Aiken and D. Mechanic. New Brunswick, NJ: Rutgers University Press, 1987.

Friedman, Emily. "The Uninsured: From Dilemma to Crisis." *Journal of the American Medical Association* 265: 2491–2495, 1991.

Friedman, Milton. *Capitalism and Freedom*. Chicago: University of Chicago Press, 1962.

Friss, Lois. "Nursing Studies Laid End to End Form a Circle." *Journal of Health Politics, Policy, and Law* 19: 597–631, 1994.

Fuchs, V. *Who Shall Live? Health, Economics and Social Choice*. New York: Basic Books, 1974.

Gay, G., J.J. Kronenfeld, S. Baker, and R. Amidon. "An Appraisal of Organizational Response to Fiscally Constraining Regulation." *Journal of Health and Social Behavior* 30: 41–55, 1989.

Gibson, R.M., and D.R. Waldo. "National Health Expenditures, 1980." *Health Care Financing Review* 3: 1–54, 1981.

Ginzberg, Eli, ed. *Regionalization and Health Policy*. Washington, DC: U.S. Government Printing Office, 1977.

GMENAC. *Report of the Graduate Medical Education National Advisory Committee to the Secretary, DHHS* (Report No. [HRA] 81–653). Washington, DC: U.S. Department of Health and Human Services, 1980.

Grumbach, Kevin, and Thomas Bodenheimer. "The Organization of Health Care." *Journal of the American Medical Association* 273: 160–167, 1995.

Guterman, S., and A. Dobson. "Impact of the Medicare Prospective Payment System For Hospitals." *Health Care Financing Review* 7: 97–114, 1986.

Haglund, Claudia, and William Dowling. "The Hospital." In *Introduction to Health Services,* 4th ed., edited by Stephen J. Williams and Paul R. Torrens. Albany, NY: Delmar, 1993.

Haglund, C., and W.L. Dowling. "The Hospital." In *Introduction to Health Services*, 3rd ed., edited by S. Williams and P. R. Torrens. New York: John Wiley and Sons, Inc., 1984.

Halvorson, George C. "An HMO Chief Executive Officer on Medicaid Managed Care." *Health Affairs* 15: 170–171, 1996.

Harvey, L.K. and S.C. Shubat. *Physician Opinion on Health Care Issues.* Chicago: American Medical Association, 1990.

Haug, Marie. "The Erosion of Professional Authority: A Cross-Cultural Inquiry in the Case of the Physician." *Milbank Memorial Fund Quarterly* 54: 83–106, 1976.

Haug, Marie. "A Reexamination of the Hypothesis of Physician Deprofessionalization." *Milbank Quarterly* 66 (suppl.): 48–56, 1988.

Havighurst, Craig. "HMO Phobia: Who's Afraid of Managed Care Mergers?" *Healthcare Leadership Review* 15: 4, 1996.

Health Insurance Association of America. *Source Book of Health Insurance Data, 1990.* Washington, DC: Health Insurance Association of America, 1990.

Health-PAC. *The American Health Empire: Power, Profits and Politics*. New York: Vintage, 1970.

Heclo, Hugh. "The Clinton Health Plan: Historical Perspectives." *Health Affairs* 14: 86–98, 1995.

Hefler, Stephen K., Carolyn S. Donham, Darleen K. Won, and Arthur L. Sensenig. "Health Care Indicators: Hospital, Employment and Price Indicators for the Health Care Industry." *Health Care Financing Review* 17: 217–256, 1996.

Himmelfarb, Richard. *Catastrophic Politics: The Rise and Fall of the Medicare Catastrophic Coverage Act of 1988*. University Park, PA: Pennsylvania State University Press, 1995.

Hospital Statistics. Chicago: American Hospital Association, 1991.

Hoy, E.W., R.E. Curtis, and T. Rice. "Change and Growth in Managed Care." *Health Affairs* 10: 18–36, 1991.

Hsiao, W.C., D.B. Yntema, P. Braun, and E. Becker. "Resource Based Relative Values: An Overview." *Journal of the American Medical Association* 260: 2347–2353, 1988.

Jacobs, Lawrence. "Health Reform Impasse: The Politics of American Ambivalence Toward Government." *Journal of Health Politics, Policy and Law* 18: 629–655, 1993.

Jecker, Nancy S. "Employer-Based Insurance." In *The Politics of Health Care Reform*, edited by James A. Morone and Gary S. Belkin. Durham, NC: Duke University Press, 1994.

Jensen, Joyce. "HMO Satisfaction Slipping." *Modern Healthcare*, pp. 86–88, October 7, 1996.

Johnson, Haynes, and David S. Broder. *The System: The American Way of Politics at the Breaking Point*. Boston: Little, Brown and Company, 1996.

Jonas, S. *An Introduction to the U.S. Health Care System*, 3rd ed. New York: Springer, 1992.

Kaluzny, Arnold, and Stephen Shortell. "Creating and Managing the Future." In *Essentials of Health Care Management*, edited by Stephen Shortell and Arnold Kaluzny. Albany, NY: Delmar Publishers, 1997.

Kasper, J.D. "The Importance of Type of Children's Usual Source of Care for Children's Physician Expenditures and Access." *Medical Care* 25: 386–398, 1987.

Kertesz, Louise. "HMO Enrollment Soars, Profits Don't." *Modern Healthcare*, p. 10, October 28, 1996.

Kingdon, John W. *Agendas, Alternatives and Public Policies*. Boston: Little, Brown and Company, 1984.

Kleinman, J.D., M. Gold, and D. Makuc. "Use of Ambulatory Medical Care by the Poor." *Medical Care* 19: 1011–1022, 1981.

Koch, A.L. "Financing Health Services." In *Introduction to Health Services*, edited by J. Williams and P.R. Torrens. New York: John Wiley and Sons, 1988.

Kronenfeld, Jennie Jacobs. *Controversial Issues in Health Care Policy*. Newbury Park, CA: Sage Publications, 1993.

Kronenfeld, Jennie Jacobs. "Sources of Ambulatory Care and Utlization Models." *Health Services Research* 15: 3–20, 1980.

Kronenfeld, Jennie Jacobs, and Marcia Lynn Whicker. *Captive Populations: Caring for the Young, the Sick, the Imprisoned, and the Elderly*. New York: Praeger, 1990.

Kronenfeld, Jennie Jacobs and Marcia Lynn Whicker. *U.S. National Health Policy: An Analysis of the Federal Role*. New York: Praeger, 1984.

Kutner, N.G. "Cost-Benefit Issues in U.S. National Health Legislation: The Case of the End Stage Renal Disease Program." *Social Problems* 30: 51–64, 1982.

Kutner, N.G. "Issues in the Application of High Cost Medical Technology: The Case of Organ Transplantation." In *The Sociology of Health and Illness: Critical Perspectives*, edited by P. Conrad and R. Kern. New York: St. Martin's Press, 1990.

Landerfeld, J.S., and R.P. Parker. "Review of the Comprehensive Revision of the National Income and Product Accounts." *Survey of Current Business*. Washington, DC: U.S. Government Printing Office, 1995.

Lazerby, Helen C., and S.W. Letsch. "National Health Expenditures, 1989." *Health Care Financing Review* 12: 1–26, 1990.

Leape, Lucian L. "Unnecessary Surgery." *Annual Review of Public Health* 13: 363–383, 1992.

Lee, Phillip R., and A.E. Benjamin. "Health Policy and the Politics of Health Care." In *Introduction to Health Services*, 4th ed., edited by Stephen J. Williams and Paul R. Torrens. Albany, NY: Delmar, 1993.

Levit, Katherine R., H.C. Lazerby, S.W. Letsch, and Cathy A. Cowan, "National Health Care Spending, 1989." *Health Affairs* 10: 117–139, 1991a.

Levit, Katherine R., Helen C. Lazerby, and Lekha Sivarajan. "Health Care Spending in 1994: Slowest in Decades." *Health Affairs* 15: 130–144, 1996a.

Levit, Katherine R., Helen C. Lazerby, Cathy A. Cowan, and S.W. Letsch. "National Health Care Expenditures, 1990." *Health Care Financing Review* 13: 29–54, 1991b.

Levit, Katherine R., Helen C. Lazerby, Lekha Sivarajan, Madle Stewart, Bradley Braden, Charles C. Cowan, Carolyn S. Donham, Anna M. Long, Patricia A. McDonnell, Arthur L. Sensenig, Jean M. Stiller, and Darleen K. Won. "National Health Expenditures, 1994." *Health Care Financing Review* 17: 205–261, 1996b.

Lindblom, C.E. "The Science of Muddling Through." *Public Administration Review* 14: 79–88, 1959.

Longest, Beaufort B., Jr. *Health Policymaking in the United States.* Ann Arbor, MI: AUPHA Press, 1994.

Lucas, Deborah. "Managed Competition with Prefunding: The Solution for Long-Term Care." *Milbank Quarterly* 74: 571–597, 1996.

Luft, Harold. *Health Maintenance Organizations.* New York: John Wiley and Sons, Inc., 1981.

Luft, Harold S., and Merwyn R. Greenlick. "The Contribution of Group and Staff-Model HMOs to American Medicine." *Milbank Quarterly* 74: 445–467, 1996.

Lumsdon, Kevin. "Beyond Four Walls." *Hospitals and Health Networks*, pp. 44–45, March 5, 1994.

Lynch, Thomas D. *Public Budgeting in America.* Englewood Cliffs, NJ: Prentice-Hall, 1979.

McIlrath, Sharon. "HCFA Issues Final RBRVS Rules." *American Medical News*, pp. 1, 26–47, December 1991a.

McIlrath, Sharon. "RBRVS Launch Could Be Difficult." *American Medical News*, pp. 1, 37, December 1991b.

McIlrath, Sharon "New Restrictions on HMOs." *American Medical News*, pp. 1, 31, December 2, 1996.

McKinlay, J., and J. Stoeckle, "Corporatization and the Social Transformation of Doctoring." In *The Sociology Of Health and Illness: Critical Perspectives*, edited by P. Conrad and R. Kern. New York: St. Martin's Press, 1989.

Macridis, Roy C. *Contemporary Political Ideologies: Movements and Regimes*, 2nd ed. Boston: Little, Brown and Company, 1983.

Manderscheid, R.W., and M.A. Sonnenschein, eds. *Mental Health, United States, 1990.* DHHD Publication No. (ADM) 90–178. Washington, DC: U.S. Government Printing Office, 1990.

Mayer, D. "Limited Class Size at Nursing Schools Baffles Hospitals." *Health Week*, pp. 1, 31, October 21, 1991.

Mechanic, David, and David Rochefort. "Deinstitutionalizaton: An Appraisal of Reform." *Annual Review of Sociology* 16: 301–327, 1990.

"Medicap Reforms Making It Easier for Customers to Know What They Are Buying." *Health Care Financing and Organization News and Progress.* Washington, DC: Alpha Center, pp. 4–5, November 1996.

Menken, Matthew. "Caring for the Underserved: Health Insurance Coverage Is Not Enough." *Caring for the Uninsured and Underinsured.* Chicago: American Medical Association, 1991.

Mick, Stephen S., and Ira Moscovice. "Health Care Professionals." In *Introduction to Health Services,* 4th ed., edited by Stephen J. Williams and Paul R. Torrens. Albany, NY: Delmar, 1993.

Moccia, P. "Toward the Future: How Could 2 Million Registered Nurses Not Be Enough?" *Nursing Clinics of North America* 25: 605–613, 1990.

Moffitt, G. Kevin, Pamela B. Daly, Lisa Tracey, Mitchell Galloway, and Thomas C. Tinstman. "Patient-Focused Care: Key Principles to Restructuring." *Hospital and Health Services Administration* 38: 509–521, 1995.

Montague, Jim. "Currents." *Hospitals and Health Networks,* p. 12, September 20, 1996.

Morrisey, J.P., H.H. Goldman, and L.V. Klerman. "Cycles of Institutional Reform." In *Mental Health Care and Social Policy*, edited by P. Brown. Boston: Routledge and Kegan Paul, pp. 70–98, 1985.

Moscovice, I. "Health Care Professionals." In *Introduction to Health Services*, edited by S.J. Williams and R.R. Torrens. New York: John Wiley and Sons, Inc, 1988.

Mowell, Charles A. "The Search for Solutions to the Indigent Care Crisis." *Health Care Financial Management*, pp. 19–25, August 1989.

Moyer, M. Eugene. "A Revised Look at the Number of Uninsured Americans." *Health Affairs* 8: 102–110, Summer 1989.

Mullan, F. "Poor People, Poor Policy." *Health Affairs* 6: 113–117, Spring 1987.

National Center for Health Statistics. *Health Resources Statistics.* Washington, DC: U. S. Government Printing Office, 1971.

Navarro, Vincente. *The Politics of Health Policy: The U.S. Reforms, 1980–1994.* Cambridge, MA: Blackwell Publishers, 1994.

Newschaffer, C.J., and J.A. Schoenman. "Registered Nurse Shortages: The Road to Appropriate Public Policy." *Health Affairs* 9: 98–106, 1990.

"Nursing School Enrollments Up." *American Medical World News*, p. 8, January 17, 1992.

Office of National Cost Estimates. "National Health Expenditures, 1988." *Health Care Financing Review* 11: 1–54, 1990.

Page, Leigh. "Western Voters Face Variety of Health-Related Initiatives." *American Medical News*, p. 7, October 21, 1996.

Pepper Commission. U.S. Bipartisan Commission on Comprehensive Health Care. *A Call For Action.* Washington, DC: U.S. Government Printing Office, 1990.

Petersdorf, R.G. "Primary Care Applicants—They Get No Respect." *New England Journal of Medicine* 326: 408–409, 1992.

Peterson, Mark A. "Political Influence in the 1990s: From Iron Triangles to Policy Networks." *Journal of Health Politics, Policy, and Law* 18: 395–438, 1993.

Pew Health Professions Commission. *Shifting the Supply of Our Health Care Workforce: A Guide to Redirecting Federal Subsidy of Medical Education.* San Francisco: University of California San Francisco, 1995.

Plough, A.L. *Borrowed Time: Artificial Organs and The Politics of Extending Lives.* Philadelphia: Temple University Press, 1986.

Porter-O'Grady, Tim. "Managing Along the Continuum: A New Paradigm for the Clinical Manager." *Nursing Adminstration Quarterly* 19: 1–12, 1995.

President's Commission for the Study of Ethical Problems in Medical and Biomedical and Behavioral Research. *Report: The Ethical Implications of Differences in the Availability of Health Services.* Washington, DC: March 1983.

Raffel, Marshall W. *The U.S. Health System: Origins and Functions.* New York: John Wiley and Sons, 1980.

Reagan, M.D. *The New Federalism.* New York: Oxford University Press, 1972.

Reinhardt, Uwe E. "Breaking American Health Policy Gridlock." *Health Affairs* 10: 96–103, 1991.

Reverby, S.A. "Caring Dilemma: Womanhood and Nursing in Historical Perspective." In *The Sociology Of Health and Illness: Critical Perspectives,* edited by P. Conrad and R. Kern. New York: St. Martin's Press, 1990.

Rice, Thomas H. "Containing Health Care Costs." In *Changing the U.S. Health Care Delivery System,* edited by Ronald M. Andersen, Thomas H. Rice, and Gerald F. Kominski. San Francisco: Jossey-Bass Publishers, 1996.

Rimlinger, Gaston. *Welfare Policy and Industrialization in Europe, America, and Russia.* New York: Wiley, 1971.

Robinson, James C. "The Changing Boundaries of the American Hospital." *The Milbank Quarterly* 72: 259–268, 1994.

Rosenberg, C.E. *The Care of Strangers: The Rise of the American Hospital System.* New York: Basic Books, 1987.

Rosenstiel, Thomas. "Press Found Putting Stress on Politics of Health Reform." *Los Angeles Times* A24, March 26, 1994.

Ruttenberg, Joan E. "Revisiting the Employer-Insurance Link." In *The Politics of Health Care Reform,* edited by James A. Morone and Gary S. Belkin. Durham, NC: Duke University Press, 1994.

Salkever, D.S. and T.W. Bice. *Hospital Certificate of Need Controls: Impact on Investment, Cost, and Need.* Washington, DC: American Enterprise Institute for Public Policy Research, 1979.

Schieber, G.J., J.P. Poullier, and L.M. Greenwald. "U.S. Health Expenditure Performance: An International Comparison and Data Update." *Health Care Financing Review* 13: 1–87, 1992.

Schroeder, Steven A. "How Can We Tell Whether There Are Too Many or Too Few Physicians? The Case for Benchmarking." *Journal of the American Medical Association* 276: 1841–1844, 1996.

Sensenig, Arthur L., Stephen K. Heffler, and Carolyn S. Donham. "Health Care Indicators." *Health Care Financing Review* 17: 269–306, 1996.

Service, Mary. "Why Health Costs Got Smaller in 1994." *Business and Health,* pp. 20–28, March 1995.

Shonick, William. "Public Health Agencies and Services: The Partnership Network." In *Introduction to Health Services,* 4th ed., edited by Stephen J. Williams and Paul R. Torrens. Albany, NY: Delmar, 1993.

Shortell, Stephen M., Robin R. Gillies, and David Anderson. "The New World of Managed Care: Creating Organized Delivery Systems." *Health Affairs* 13: 46–64, 1994.

Shortell, Stephen M., Robin R. Gillies, and Kelly J. Devers. "Reinventing the American Hospital." *The Milbank Quarterly* 73: 131–160, 1995.

Siu, A.L., F.A. Sonnenberg, W.G. Manning, G.A. Goldberg, E.S. Blumfield, J.P. Newhouse, and R.H. Brooke. "Inappropriate Use of Hospitals in a Randomized Trial of Health Insurance Plans." *New England Journal of Medicine* 315: 1259–1266, 1986.

Skopcol, Theda. "Is the Time Finally Ripe?: Health Insurance Reforms in the 1990s." In *The Politics of Health Care Reform: Lessons from the Past, Prospects for the Future*, edited by James A. Morone and Gary S. Belkin. Durham, NC: Duke University Press, 1994.

Skopcol, Theda. *Protecting Soldiers and Mothers: The Political Origins of Social Policy in the United States*. Cambridge, MA: Harvard University Press, 1992.

Skopcol, Theda. "The Rise and Resounding Demise of the Clinton Plan." *Health Affairs* 14: 66–85, 1995.

Starr, Paul. *The Logic of Health Care Reform*. New York: Penguin Books, 1994.

Starr, Paul. "The Middle Class and National Health Care Reform." *American Prospect* 12: 44–52, 1991.

Starr, Paul. *The Social Transformation of American Medicine*. New York: Basic Books, 1982.

"The State of Health Care in America." *Business and Health* 13 (suppl. C): 1995.

Steinmo, Sven, and Jon Watts. "It's the Institutions, Stupid! Why Comprehensive National Health Insurance Always Fails in America." *Journal of Health Politics, Policy and Law* 20: 329–371, 1995.

Stelzer, I.M. "There Is No Health Care Crisis." *Wall Street Journal*, Section A, p. 12, January 25, 1994.

Stevens, Beth. "Blurring the Boundaries: How the Federal Government has Influenced Welfare Benefits in the Private Sector." In *The Politics of Social Policy in the United States*, edited by Margaret Weir, Ann Shola Orloff, and Theda Skopcol. Princeton, NJ: Princeton Universtiy Press, 1988.

Stevens, Rosemary. *American Medicine and the Public Interest*. New Haven, CT: Yale University Press, 1971.

Stevens, R. *In Sickness and in Wealth: American Hospitals in the Twentieth Century*. New York: Basic Books, 1989.

Stevenson, Richard W. "Sharp Differences and Compromise Are Likely on Budget." *The New York Times*, p. 12, January 12, 1997.

Stoeckle, John D. "The Citadel Cannot Hold: Technologies Go Outside the Hospital, Patients and Doctors Too." *Milbank Quarterly* 73: 131–160, 1995.

Strickland, Stephen. *Research and the Health Of Americans: Improving the Public Policy Process*. Lexington, MA: Lexington Books, 1978.

Thompson, Robert S. "What Have HMOs Learned About Clinical Prevention Services?" *Milbank Quarterly* 74: 469–509, 1996.

Thorpe, Kenneth E. "The Best of Both Worlds: Merging Competition and Regulation." *Journal of American Health Policy*, pp. 20–24, July/August 1992.

Todd, James S., Steven V. Seekins, Johan A. Kirchbaum, and Lynn Harvey. "Health Access in America—Strengthening the U.S. Health Care System." *Journal of the American Medical Association* 265: 2503–2506, 1991.

Toner, Robin. "Harry and Louise Were Right, Sort Of." *The New York Times*, Section 4, Editorials and Op-Ed, pp. 1, 3, November 24, 1996.

Torrens, Paul R. "Historical Evolution and Overview of Health Services in the United States." In *Introduction to Health Services*, 4th ed., edited by Stephen J. Williams and Paul R. Torrens. Albany, NY: Delmar, 1993.

Torrens, Paul R., and Stephen J. Williams. "Understanding the Present, Planning for the Future: The Dynamics of Health Care in the United States in the 1990s." In *Introduction to Health Services*, 4th ed., edited by Stephen J. Williams and Paul R. Torrens. Albany, NY: Delmar, 1993.

U.S. Bureau of the Census. *Current Population Survey*. Washington, DC: 1986.

U.S. Department of Health and Human Services, Steering Commmittee on the Chronically Mentally Ill. *Toward a National Plan for the Chronically Mentally Ill*. Washington, DC: U.S. Government Printing Office, 1980.

Updated Report on Access to Health Care for the American People. Special Report Number 1. Princeton, NJ: Robert Wood Johnson Foundation, 1983.

Verhoven, Sam Howe. "Legislators Meet, Surprised at Limit on Shift of Power." *The New York Times*, pp. 1, 12, January 12, 1997.

Votz, D. and J.D. Cochrane. "The Future of Provider-Sponsored HMOs." *Integrated Health Report*, pp. 1–9, August 1996.

Waldo, D.R., K.R. Levit, and H. Lazerby. "National Health Expenditures, 1985." *Health Care Financing Review* 8: 1–21, 1986.

Wallace, Helen, Edwin M. Gold, and Allan C. Oglesby. *Maternal and Child Health Practices: Problems, Resources, and Methods of Delivery*, 2nd. ed. New York: John Wiley and Sons, 1982.

Wallace, Steven P., Emily K. Abel, and Pamela Stefanowicz. "Long-Term Care and the Elderly." In *Changing the U.S. Health Care Delivery System*, edited by Ronald M. Andersen, Thomas H. Rice, and Gerald F. Kominski. San Francisco: Jossey-Bass Publishers, 1996.

Warren, Kenneth F. *Adminstrative Law in the American Political System*. St. Paul, MN: West, 1982.

Weber, Max. *The Protestant Ethic and the Spirit of Capitalism*. Translated by Talcott Parsons. New York: Charles Scribner's Sons, 1958.

Weitz, Rose. *The Sociology of Health, Illness and Health Care: A Critical Approach*. Belmont, CA: Wadsworth Publishing Co., 1996.

West, Daniel M., Diane Heith, and Chris Goodwin. "Harry & Louise Go to Washington." *Journal of Health Politics, Policy and Law* 21: 35–68, 1996.

Wildavsky, Aaron. *The Politics of the Budgetary Process*. Boston: Little, Brown and Company, 1964.

Wilensky, G.R. "Viable Strategies for Dealing with the Uninsured." *Health Affairs* 6: 33–40, 1987.

Wilensky, G.R., and K.E. Ladenheim. "The Uninsured." *Frontiers of Health Services Management* 4: 3–31, Winter 1987.

Williams, Stephen J. and Paul R. Torrens. "Influencing, Regulating, and Monitoring the Health Care System." In *Introduction to Health Services*, 4th ed., edited by Stephen J. Williams and Paul R. Torrens. Albany, NY: Delmar, 1993a.

Williams, Stephen J. and Paul R. Torrens. "Managed Care: Restructuring the System." In *Introduction to Health Services*, 4th ed., edited by Stephen J. Williams and Paul R. Torrens. Albany, NY: Delmar, 1993b.

Wilson, R.W., and E.L. White. "Changes in Morbidity, Disability, and Utilization Differences Between the Poor and the Nonpoor." *Medical Care* 15: 636–650, 1977.

Yankelovich, Daniel. "The Debate That Wasn't: The Public and the Clinton Plan." *Health Affairs* 14: 7–23, 1995.

Zajac, Edward J., and Thomas A. D'Aunno. "Managing Strategic Alliances." In *Essentials of Health Care Management*, edited by Stephen Shortell and Arnold Kaluzny. Albany, NY: Delmar Publishers, 1997.

SUBJECT INDEX

AUTHOR INDEX

ABOUT THE AUTHOR

JENNIE JACOBS KRONENFELD is Professor of Health Administration and Policy, Arizona State University. She is the author of seven earlier books on medical issues.

ISBN 0-275-95023-9

90000>

EAN

9 780275 950231

HARDCOVER BAR CODE